NOTES
from
YOGA TEACHER TRAINING

SKETCHNOTES *by* EVA-LOTTA LAMM

ISBN 978-3-9820693-2-6

Self-published
by Eva-Lotta Lamm, Berlin

First published in 2017
1st Edition, September 2017
6th Printing, March 2020

I FIRST MET MY TEACHER SURINDER SINGH WHEN WE
STAYED IN RISHISKESH FOR A WEEK ON OUR WORLD
TRIP IN 2014. AFTER SPENDING 1 1/2 HOURS TRYING
TO FIND THE 'GREEN HOUSE' IN JONK VILLAGE WHERE
HE IS TEACHING, WALKING THE NARROW STREETS AND
ASKING DOZENS OF PEOPLE IN THE NEIGHBORHOOD
WHERE WE WOULD FIND IT, WE ATTENDED HIS DROP-IN
CLASSES EVERY MORNING DURING OUR STAY.

EVEN BEFORE WE LEFT I DECIDED TO COME BACK AND
STUDY WITH SURINDER FOR LONGER. I SIGNED UP FOR
HIS TEACHER TRAINING COURSE AND IN OCTOBER 2016
I TRAVELLED BACK TO INDIA.

WE PRACTICED AND STUDIED ASANA, PRANAYAMA,
PHILOSOPHY, ANATOMY, CHANTING AND MEDITATION.

THIS BOOK CONTAINS MY NOTES FROM THE MONTH-
LONG HATHA YOGA TRAINING COURSE AS WELL AS FROM
SOME ADDITIONAL CLASSES I TOOK AFTER THE COURSE
FINISHED.

I'M DEEPLY GRATEFUL TO MY TEACHERS

SURINDER SINGH
VIMAL SHARMA
GURMEET SINGH
SWAMIJI ATMA
ASHISH SHARMA

FOR SHARING THEIR KNOWLEDGE
WITH PASSION AND KINDNESS.

AND TO MY BEAUTIFUL CLASSMATES
FOR MAINTAINING OUR POSES
AND HOLDING OUR SUNS TOGETHER.

THIS IS.
:)

PEOPLE - WATCHING...

DR. DRE ↘

COOL CAT

at DELHI AiRPORt with his white WiReless BEATS headphones, blue-mirrored glasses, jeans, white Sneakers & traditional white desert DRess on...

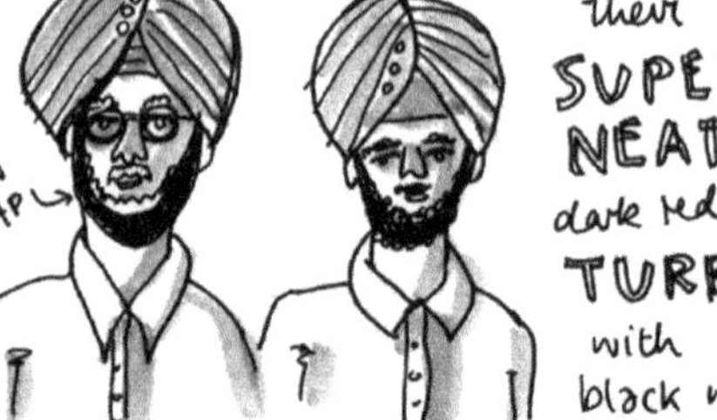

TWO GUYS on the bus to the Plane to Dehradun in their **SUPER-NEAT** dark red **TURBANS** with black netty **CHIN-STRAPS**

white plastic rings ↓

A BiG GROUP of MEN and WOMEN walking along the road between LAXMAN JHULA & RAM JHULA

=

LADIES with lots of **WHITE PLASTIC RINGS** around their upper arms. very wide at the top, getting tighter and tighter towards the elbow. (not sure how they ever get them off... ?)

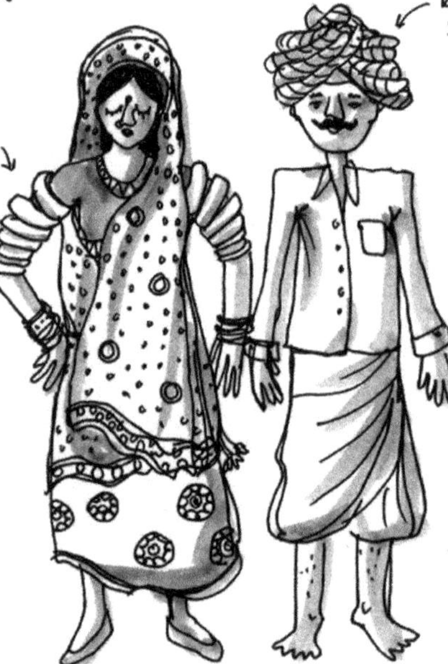

=

bright Red & super twisty ↙

MEN in white neat SHiRt & LUNGi COMBo, with just a moustache and a **TOMATO RED** super **TWISTY TURBAN**

→ very neat look!

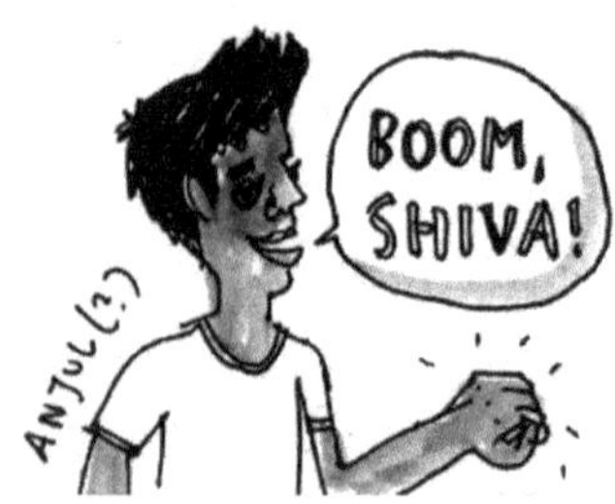

the young GUY (22?) Running BONFiRE Hostel being all happy, energetic & chatty, offering a Ghetto Fist for a greeting with a booming "BOOM SHIVA!". He Reminded me a bit of KHAN from BiKANEER, just more over the top... ☺

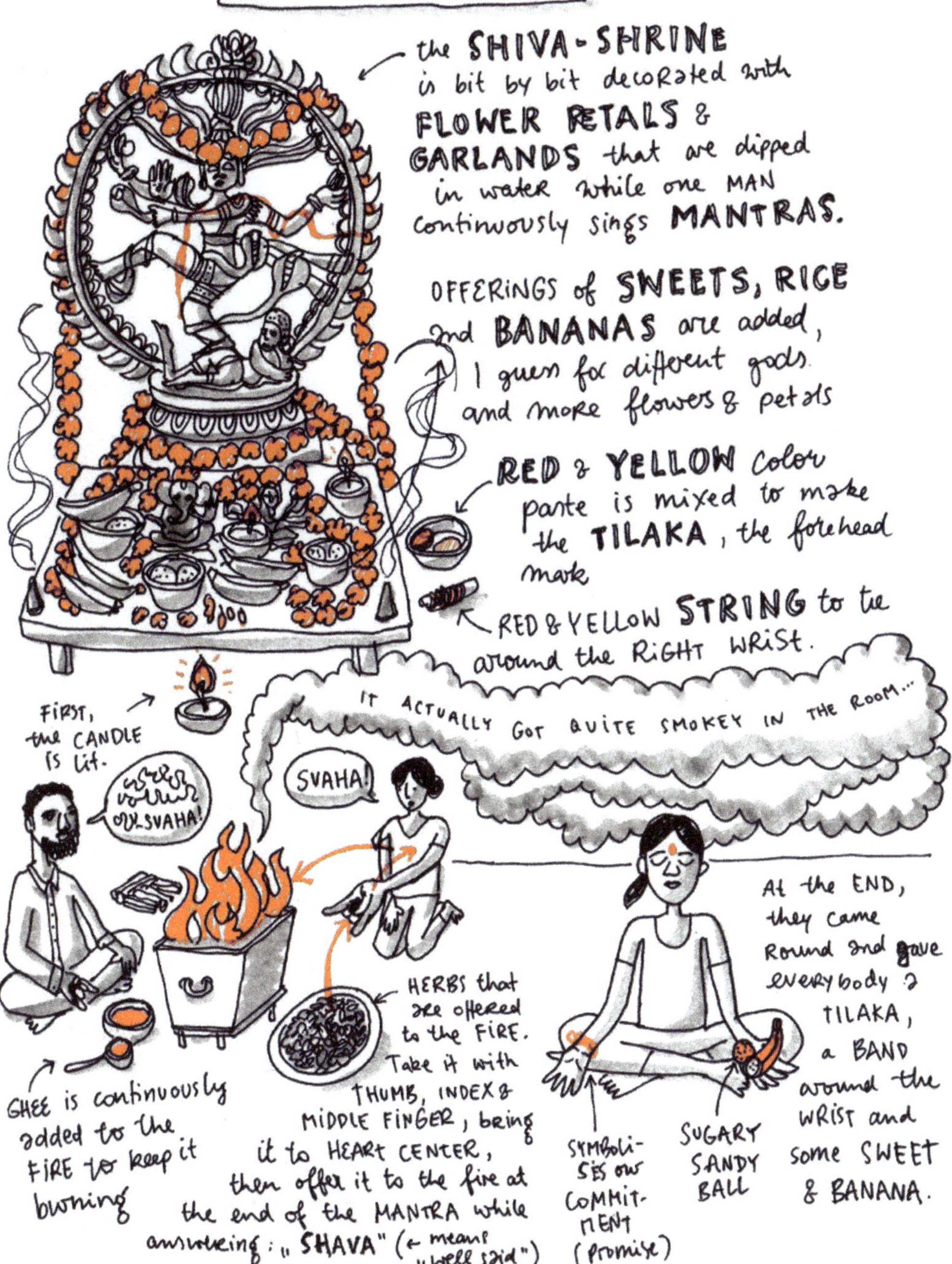

the FIRE RITUAL
07-OCT-2016
the SHIVA-SHRINE is bit by bit decorated with FLOWER PETALS & GARLANDS that are dipped in water while one MAN continuously sings MANTRAS.
OFFERINGS of SWEETS, RICE and BANANAS are added, I guess for different gods. and more flowers & petals
RED & YELLOW color paste is mixed to make the TILAKA, the forehead mark
RED & YELLOW STRING to tie around the RIGHT WRIST.
FIRST, the CANDLE is lit.
OM SVAHA!
SVAHA!
IT ACTUALLY GOT QUITE SMOKEY IN THE ROOM...
GHEE is continuously added to the FIRE to keep it burning
HERBS that are offered to the FIRE. Take it with THUMB, INDEX & MIDDLE FINGER, bring it to HEART CENTER, then offer it to the fire at the end of the MANTRA while answering: "SHAVA" (← means "well said")
At the END, they came round and gave everybody a TILAKA, a BAND around the WRIST and some SWEET & BANANA.
symbolises our COMMITMENT (promise)
SUGARY SANDY BALL

ASANA, PRANAYAMA & SATSANG

TAUGHT BY
SURINDER SINGH

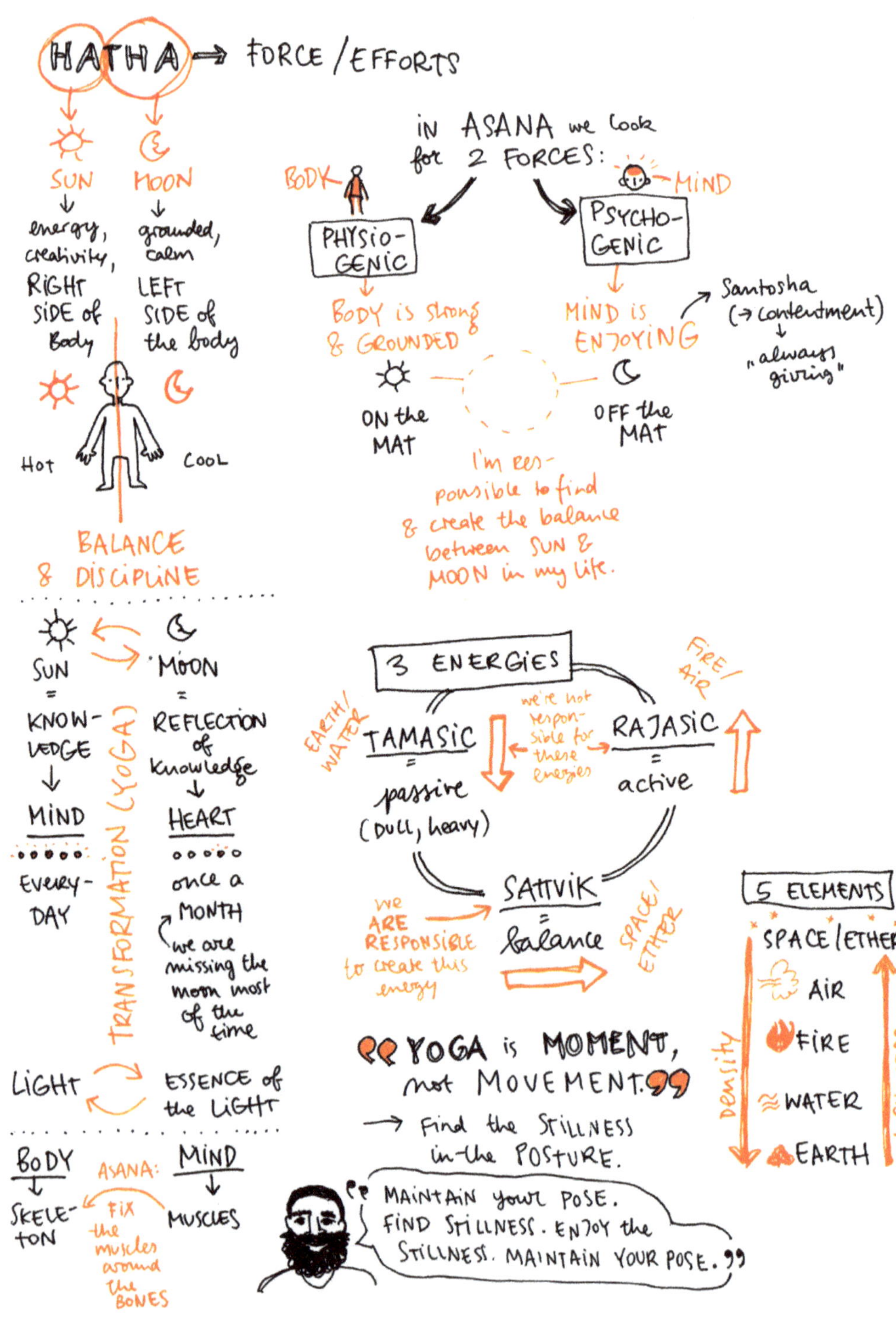

HATHA → FORCE / EFFORTS

SUN
↓
energy, creativity, RIGHT SIDE of BODY

MOON
↓
grounded, calm
LEFT SIDE of the body

Hot
Cool

BALANCE & DISCIPLINE

SUN
=
KNOWLEDGE
↓
MIND
EVERYDAY

MOON
=
REFLECTION of knowledge
↓
HEART
once a MONTH
we are missing the moon most of the time

TRANSFORMATION (YOGA)

LIGHT
ESSENCE of the LIGHT

BODY
↓
SKELETON

ASANA: fix the muscles around the bones

MIND
↓
MUSCLES

IN ASANA we look for 2 FORCES:

BODY
MIND

PHYSIO-GENIC
PSYCHO-GENIC

BODY is strong & GROUNDED
ON the MAT

MIND is ENJOYING
OFF the MAT

Santosha (→ contentment)
↓
"always giving"

I'm responsible to find & create the balance between SUN & MOON in my life.

3 ENERGIES

EARTH/WATER

TAMASIC
=
passive
(DULL, heavy)

we're not responsible for these energies

FIRE/AIR

RAJASIC
=
active

we ARE RESPONSIBLE to create this energy

SATTVIK
=
balance

SPACE/ETHER

YOGA is MOMENT, not MOVEMENT.
→ Find the STILLNESS in the POSTURE.

MAINTAIN your POSE. FIND STILLNESS. ENJOY the STILLNESS. MAINTAIN YOUR POSE.

5 ELEMENTS
SPACE/ETHER
AIR
FIRE
WATER
EARTH

density
LIGHTNESS

| 10 Oct | SURINDER'S CLASS

EXPRESS yourself
through the
GENTLENESS
of your breath

the PURPOSE of
the MIND : to understand
the BODY : to make
action
the HEART : to
express yourself

observing the
BREATH
helps us to
turn our
mind to the
INSIDE

we are so BEAUTIFUL
inside, so GENTLE, so
SOFT, we can express this
with our BREATH.

- - - - - | KAPALABATI | - - - - -

PREPARATION: ① Notice, which
nostril is
more dominant
(more open)

② BREATHE IN
through
dominant
nostril

③ BREATHE
out
through
other
nostril

~ 15-20 times, ④
then switch

SKULL SHINING
KAPALABATI (3 ROUNDS):

Relax the
face
& fore-
head.

EXHALE is ACTIVE,
pulling the navel in.

INHALE is PASSIVE.

don't exhale from
the chest. only
from the navel

⑤ OBSERVE
afterwards
is breathing
is more equal
through nostrils
(I had quite a bit
of mucus flowing
down the back of
my throat.)

keep a STEADY RHYTHM
for the whole time.
~ 150-200 STROKES per Round

AFTER:
INHALE deeply, EXHALE fully,
return to a normal breath.
→ OBSERVE your breath.
OBSERVE the stillness of the body

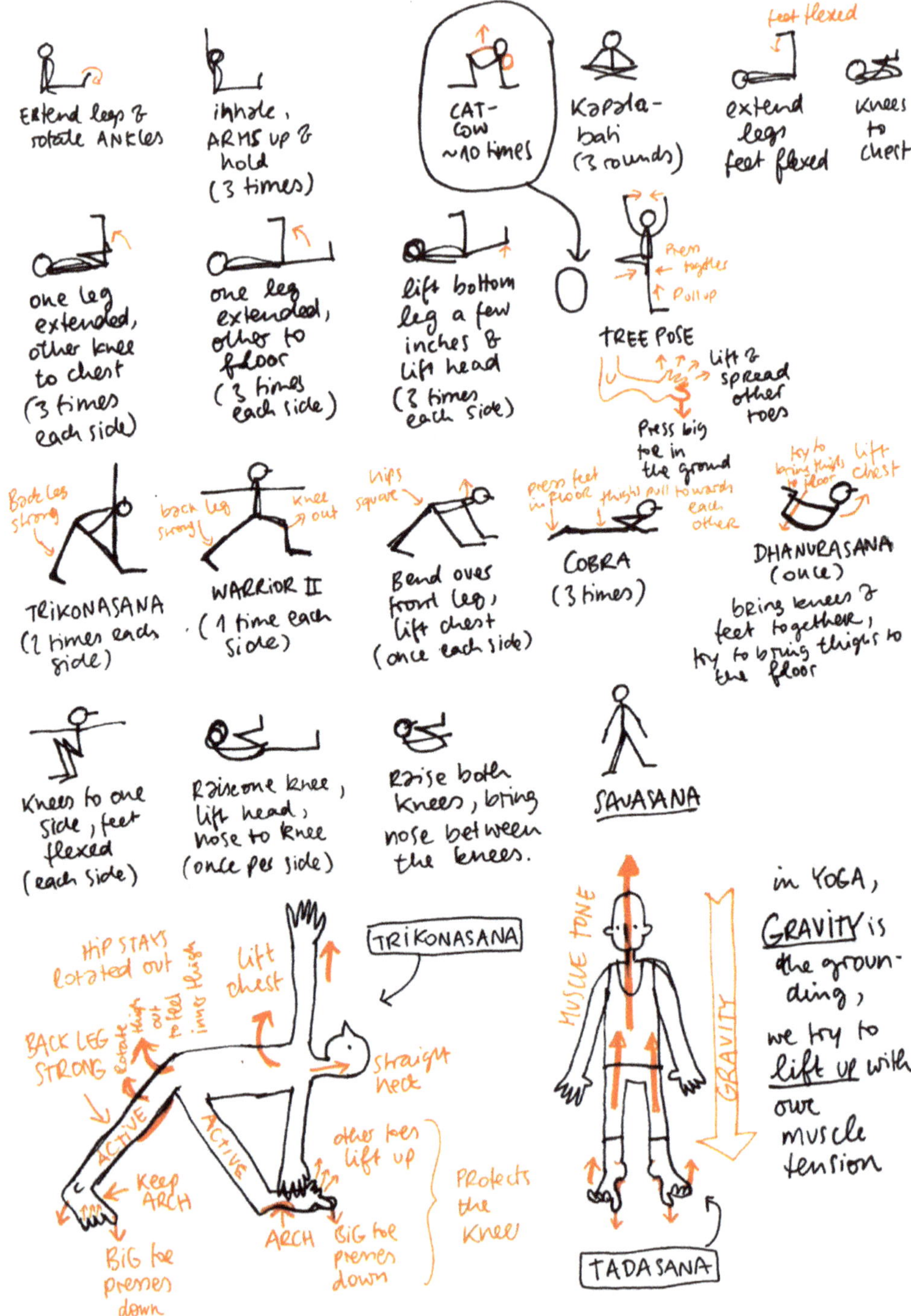

Extend legs & rotate ANKLES

inhale, ARMS up & hold (3 times)

CAT-COW ~10 times

Kapala-bati (3 rounds)

extend legs feet flexed

knees to chest

feet flexed

one leg extended, other knee to chest (3 times each side)

one leg extended, other to floor (3 times each side)

lift bottom leg a few inches & lift head (3 times each side)

TREE POSE

Press big toe in the ground

press together

pull up

Lift & spread other toes

TRIKONASANA (2 times each side)

Back leg strong

WARRIOR II (1 time each side)

back leg strong

knee out

Bend over front leg, lift chest (once each side)

hips square

COBRA (3 times)

press feet in floor

thighs pull towards each other

DHANURASANA (once)

try to bring thighs to floor

lift chest

bring knees & feet together, try to bring thighs to the floor

knees to one side, feet flexed (each side)

Raise one knee, lift head, nose to knee (once per side)

Raise both knees, bring nose between the knees.

SAVASANA

TRIKONASANA

HIP STAYS rotated out

rotate thigh out to feel inner thigh

BACK LEG STRONG

ACTIVE

ACTIVE

Lift chest

straight neck

other toes lift up

Keep ARCH

ARCH

BIG toe presses down

BIG toe presses down

PROTECTS the knee

MUSCLE TONE

GRAVITY

TADASANA

in YOGA, GRAVITY is the grounding, we try to lift up with our muscle tension

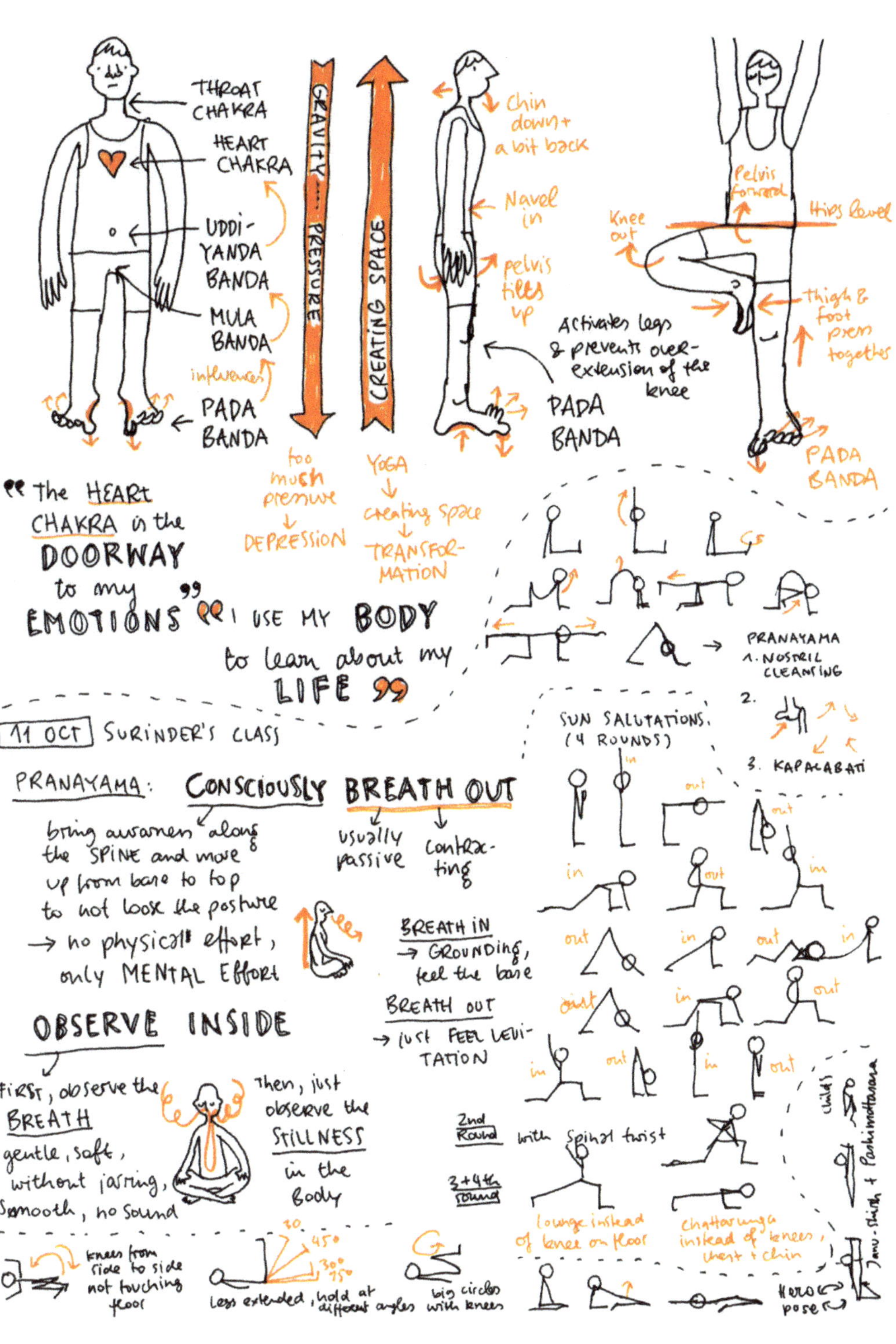

"the **HEART CHAKRA** is the **DOORWAY** to my **EMOTIONS**"

"I USE MY **BODY** to learn about my **LIFE**"

11 OCT SURINDER'S CLASS

PRANAYAMA: **CONSCIOUSLY BREATH OUT**

bring awareness along the SPINE and move up from base to top to not loose the posture → no physical effort, only MENTAL effort

usually passive   contrac-ting

BREATH IN → GROUNDING, feel the base

BREATH OUT → JUST FEEL LEVI-TATION

OBSERVE INSIDE

FIRST, observe the **BREATH**
gentle, soft, without jarring, smooth, no sound

Then, just observe the **STILLNESS** in the body

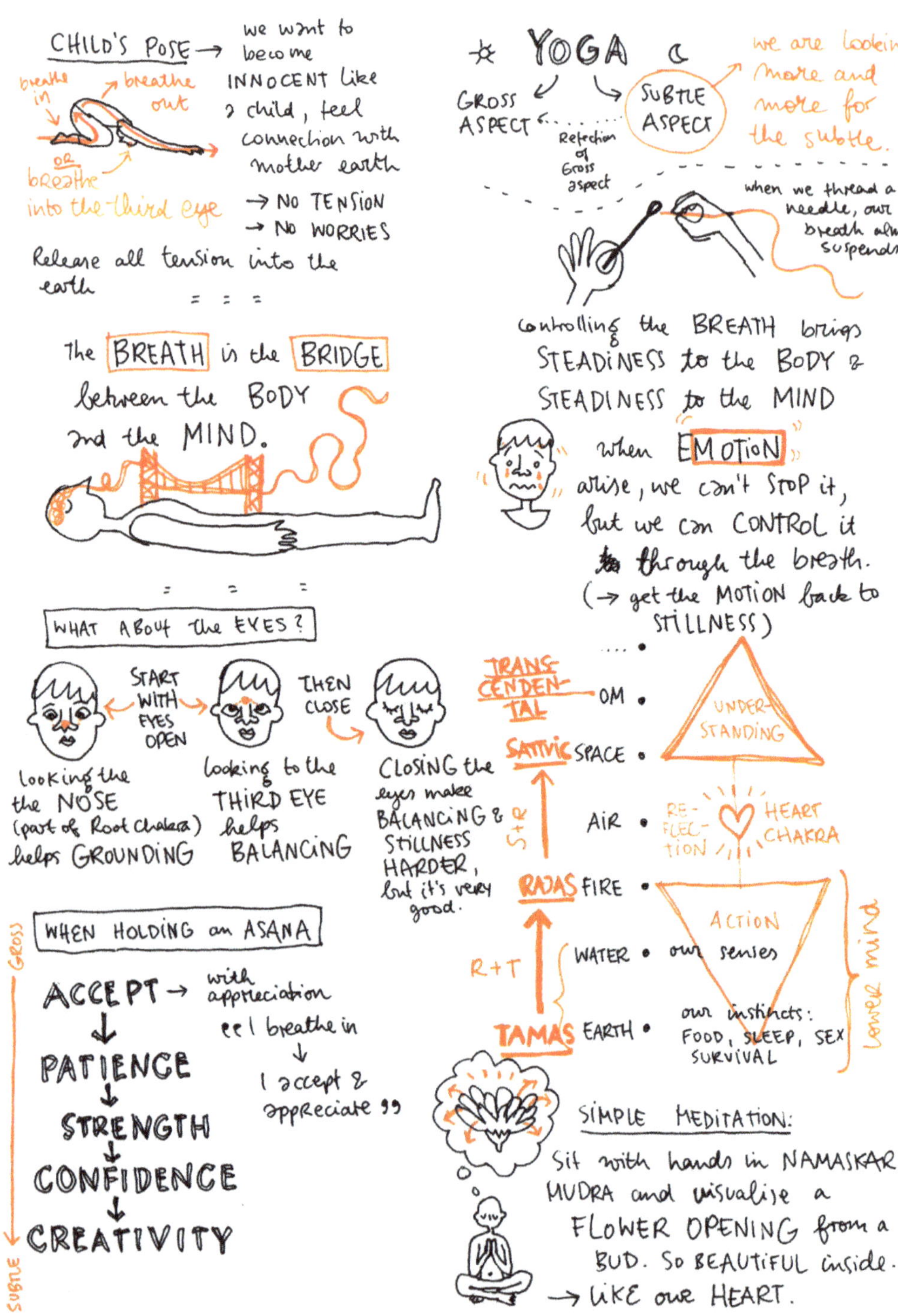

CHILD'S POSE →
breathe in
breathe out
or breathe into the third eye
we want to become INNOCENT like a child, feel connection with mother earth
→ NO TENSION
→ NO WORRIES
Release all tension into the earth

the BREATH is the BRIDGE between the BODY and the MIND.

WHAT ABOUT the EYES?
START WITH EYES OPEN
THEN CLOSE
looking the the NOSE (part of Root Chakra) helps GROUNDING
looking to the THIRD EYE helps BALANCING
CLOSING the eyes make BALANCING & STILLNESS HARDER, but it's very good.

WHEN HOLDING an ASANA
ACCEPT → with appreciation
↓
PATIENCE
↓
STRENGTH
↓
CONFIDENCE
↓
CREATIVITY
Gross
Subtle
"I breathe in
↓
I accept & appreciate"

☀ YOGA ☾
GROSS ASPECT
SUBTLE ASPECT
Reflection of Gross aspect
we are looking more and more for the subtle.
when we thread a needle, our breath almost suspends.

Controlling the BREATH brings STEADINESS to the BODY & STEADINESS to the MIND
when EMOTION arise, we can't stop it, but we can CONTROL it through the breath.
(→ get the MOTION back to STILLNESS)

TRANSCENDENTAL — OM
SATTVIC SPACE
AIR
RAJAS FIRE
WATER
TAMAS EARTH
S + R
R + T
UNDERSTANDING
REFLECTION
HEART CHAKRA
ACTION
our senses
our instincts: FOOD, SLEEP, SEX SURVIVAL
Lower mind

SIMPLE MEDITATION:
Sit with hands in NAMASKAR MUDRA and visualize a FLOWER OPENING from a BUD. SO BEAUTIFUL inside.
→ LIKE our HEART.

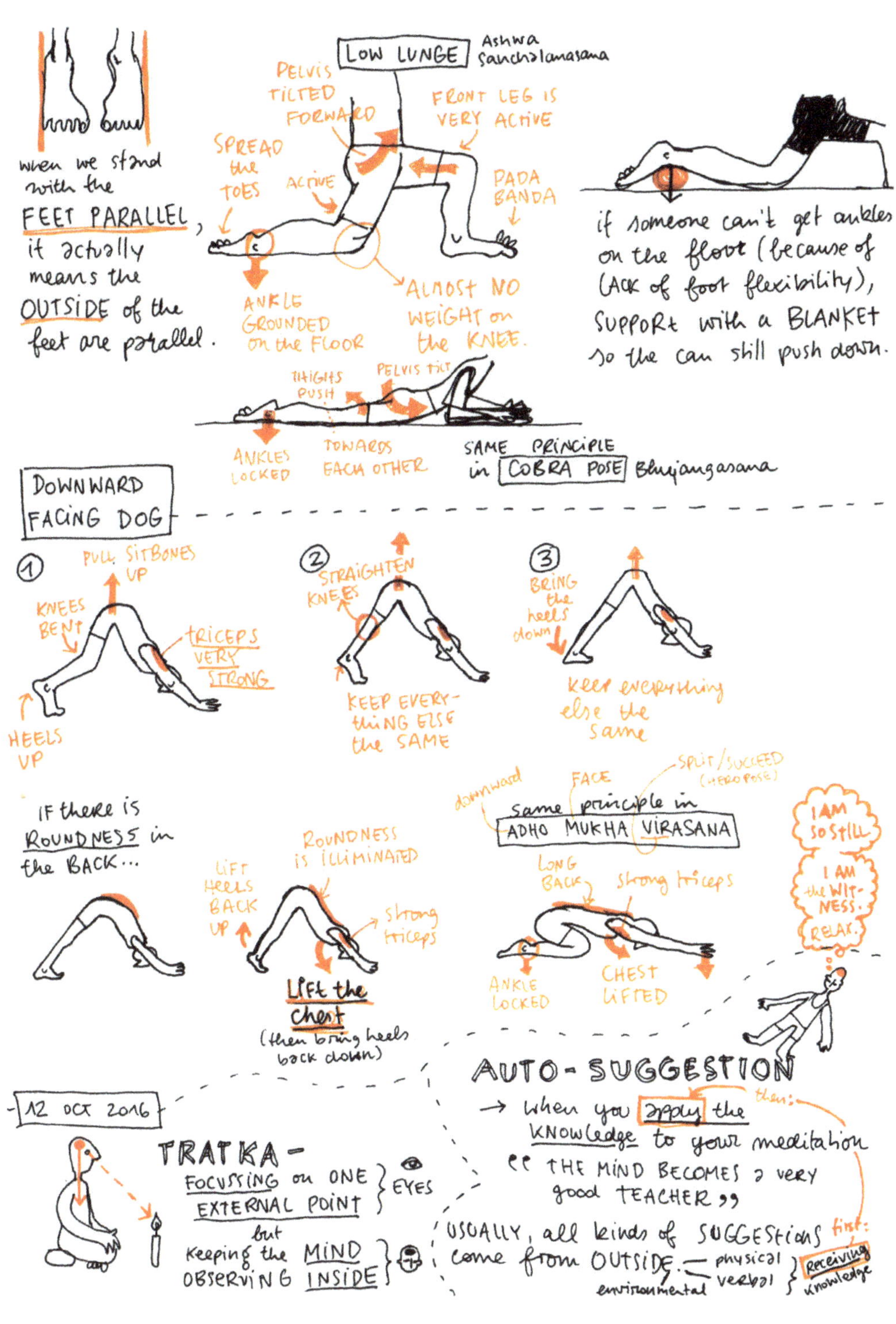

when we stand with the FEET PARALLEL, it actually means the OUTSIDE of the feet are parallel.

LOW LUNGE   Ashwa Sanchalanasana
PELVIS TILTED FORWARD
FRONT LEG IS VERY ACTIVE
SPREAD the TOES
ACTIVE
PADA BANDA
ANKLE GROUNDED ON the FLOOR
ALMOST NO WEIGHT on the KNEE.

if someone can't get ankles on the floor (because of lack of foot flexibility), SUPPORT with a BLANKET so the can still push down.

THIGHS PUSH
PELVIS tilt
ANKLES LOCKED
TOWARDS EACH OTHER
SAME PRINCIPLE in COBRA POSE Bhujangasana

DOWNWARD FACING DOG

1 PULL SITBONES UP
KNEES BENT
TRICEPS VERY STRONG
HEELS UP

2 STRAIGHTEN KNEES
KEEP EVERYTHING ELSE the SAME

3 BRING the heels down
keep everything else the same

IF there is ROUNDNESS in the BACK...

LIFT HEELS BACK UP
ROUNDNESS IS ILLIMINATED
strong triceps
LIFT the chest
(then bring heels back down)

downward FACE SPLIT/SUCCEED (HERO POSE)
same principle in ADHO MUKHA VIRASANA
LONG BACK
strong triceps
ANKLE LOCKED
CHEST LIFTED

I AM SO STILL
I AM the WITNESS.
RELAX.

AUTO-SUGGESTION
→ when you apply the KNOWLEDGE to your meditation   then:
"THE MIND BECOMES a very good TEACHER"
USUALLY, all kinds of SUGGESTIONS come from OUTSIDE.   first:
physical
environmental verbal
receiving knowledge

12 OCT 2016
TRATKA -
FOCUSSING on ONE EXTERNAL POINT } EYES
but keeping the MIND OBSERVING INSIDE

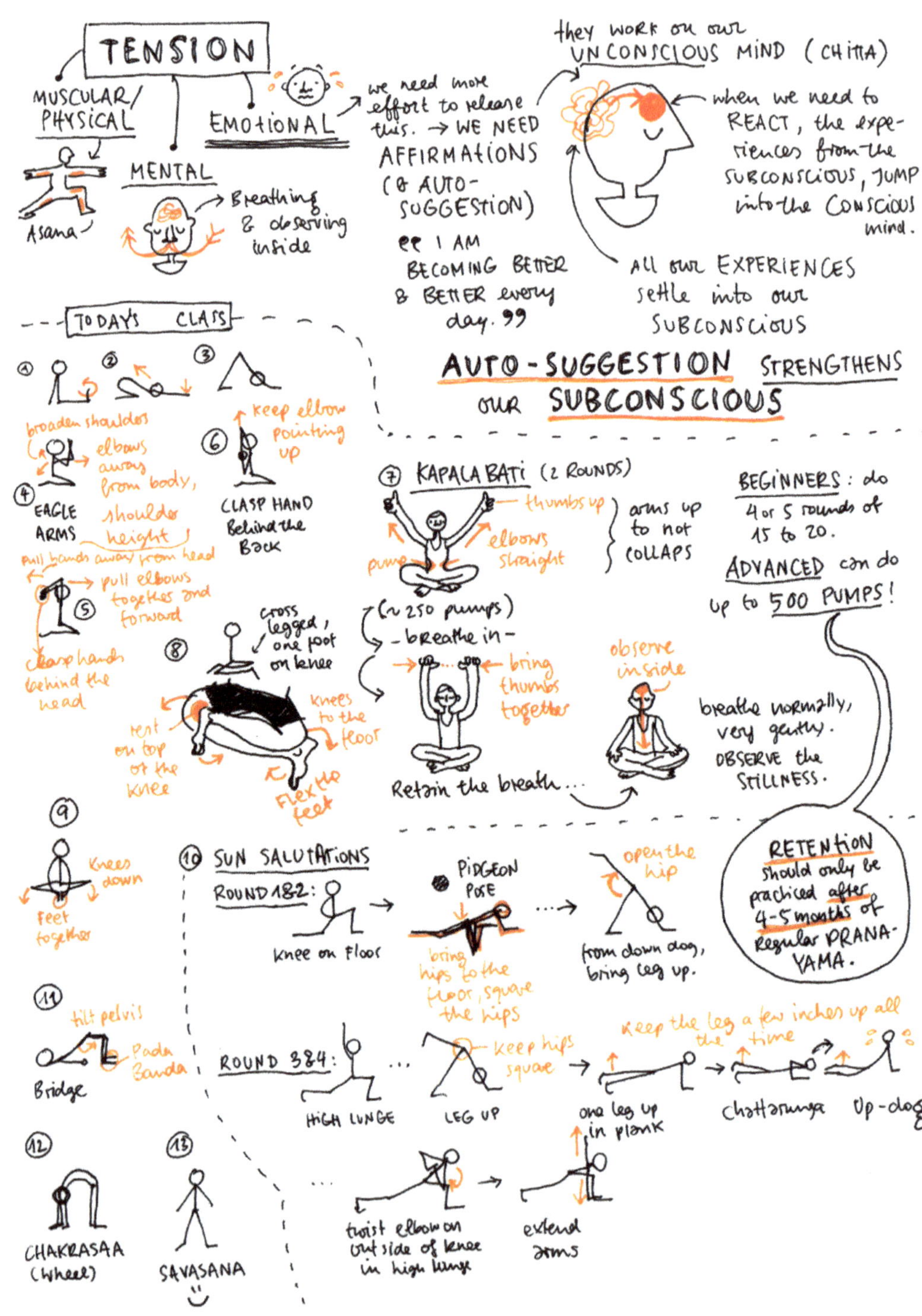

TENSION
MUSCULAR/ PHYSICAL
Asana
EMOTIONAL
MENTAL
Breathing & observing inside
we need more effort to release this. → WE NEED AFFIRMATIONS (& AUTO-SUGGESTION)
ee I AM BECOMING BETTER & BETTER every day. 99
they work on our UNCONSCIOUS MIND (CHITTA)
when we need to REACT, the experiences from the SUBCONSCIOUS, JUMP into the CONSCIOUS mind.
ALL our EXPERIENCES settle into our SUBCONSCIOUS
AUTO-SUGGESTION STRENGTHENS our SUBCONSCIOUS
TODAYS CLASS
1 2 3
broaden shoulders
elbows away from body, shoulder height
4 EAGLE ARMS
pull hands away from head
pull elbows together and forward
5
clasp hands behind the head
6 keep elbow pointing up
CLASP HAND behind the Back
cross legged, one foot on knee
8
rest on top of the knee
knees to the floor
Flex the feet
7 KAPALABATI (2 ROUNDS)
thumbs up
arms up to not COLLAPS
elbows straight
pump
(~ 250 pumps)
- breathe in -
bring thumbs together
Retain the breath...
observe inside
breathe normally, very gently. OBSERVE the STILLNESS.
BEGINNERS: do 4 or 5 rounds of 15 to 20.
ADVANCED can do up to 500 PUMPS!
RETENTION should only be practised after 4-5 months of regular PRANA-YAMA.
9 Knees down
Feet together
10 SUN SALUTATIONS
ROUND 1&2:
knee on floor
PIDGEON POSE
bring hips to the floor, square the hips
open the hip
from down dog, bring leg up.
11 tilt pelvis
Pada Bandha
Bridge
ROUND 3&4:
HIGH LUNGE
LEG UP
keep hips square
one leg up in plank
keep the leg a few inches up all the time
Chaturanga   Up-dog
12 CHAKRASAA (wheel)
13 SAVASANA
twist elbow on outside of knee in high lunge
extend arms

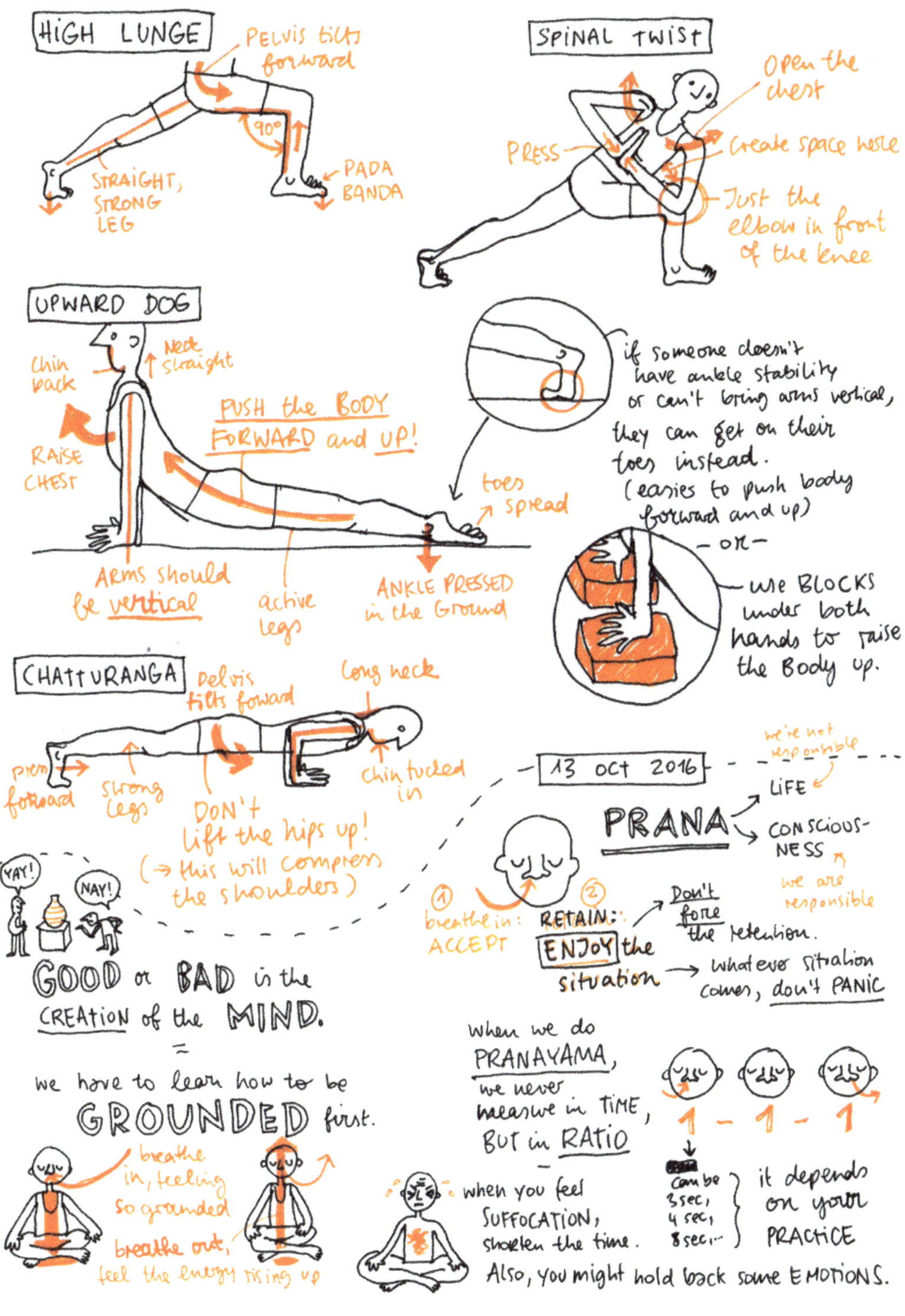
HIGH LUNGE
PELVIS tilts forward
STRAIGHT, STRONG LEG
90°
PADA BANDA

SPINAL TWIST
Open the chest
PRESS
Create space here
Just the elbow in front of the knee

UPWARD DOG
Neck straight
Chin back
RAISE CHEST
PUSH the BODY FORWARD and UP!
ARMS should be vertical
active legs
toes spread
ANKLE PRESSED in the Ground

if someone doesn't have ankle stability or can't bring arms vertical, they can get on their toes instead. (easier to push body forward and up)
— or —
use BLOCKS under both hands to raise the Body up.

CHATTURANGA
pelvis tilts foward
Long neck
press forward
strong legs
chin tucked in
DON'T lift the hips up! (→ this will compress the shoulders)

YAY!
NAY!
GOOD or BAD is the CREATION of the MIND.
=
we have to learn how to be GROUNDED first.
breathe in, feeling so grounded
breathe out, feel the energy rising up

13 OCT 2016
we're not responsible
PRANA
LIFE
CONSCIOUS-NESS
we are responsible
① breathe in: ACCEPT
② RETAIN: ENJOY the situation
Don't force the retention.
whatever situation comes, don't PANIC

when we do PRANAYAMA, we never measure in TIME, BUT in RATIO
when you feel SUFFOCATION, shorten the time.
1 - 1 - 1
can be 3 sec, 4 sec, 8 sec ...
it depends on your PRACTICE
Also, you might hold back some EMOTIONS.

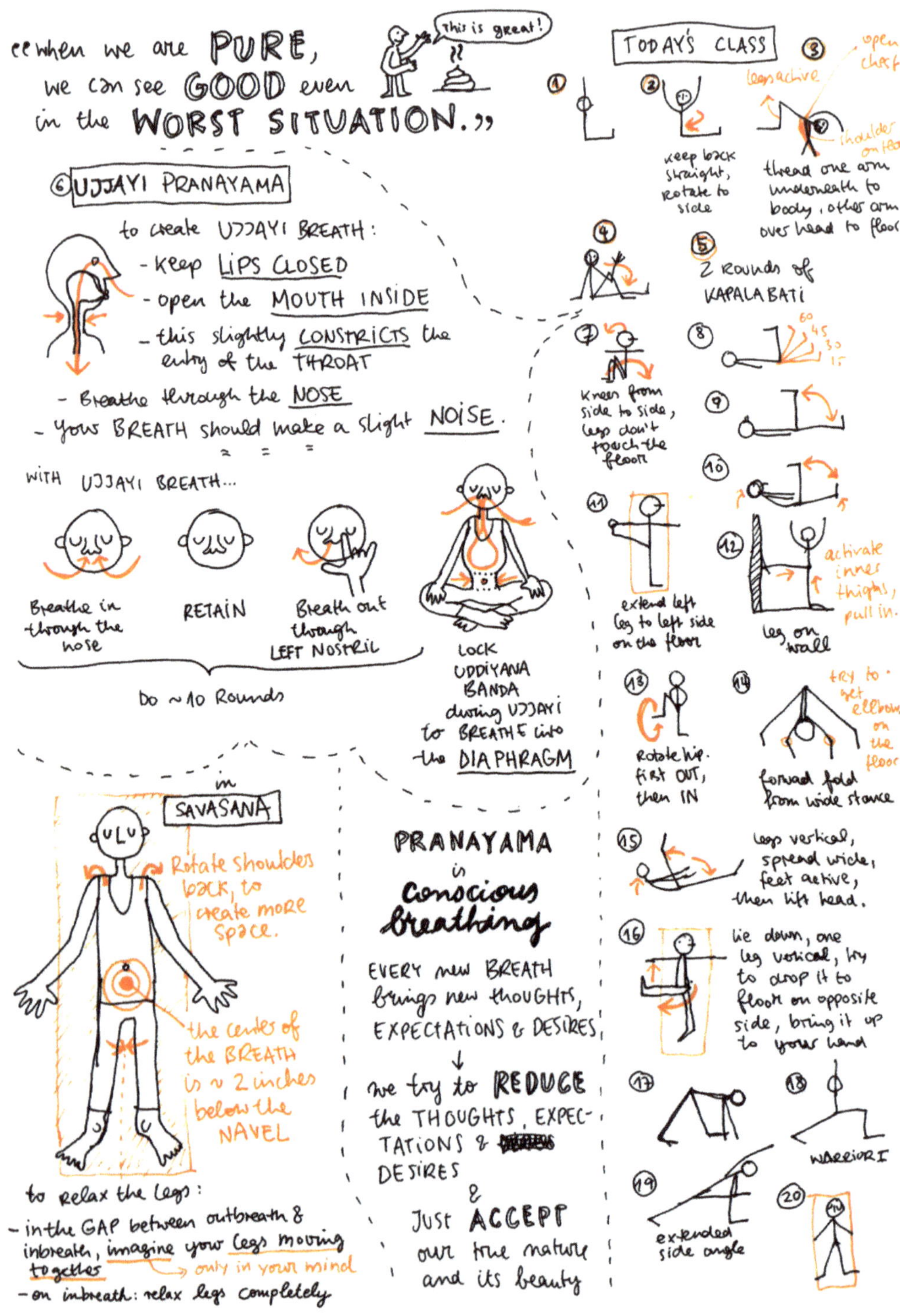

«when we are PURE, we can see GOOD even in the WORST SITUATION.»

TODAY'S CLASS

⑥ UJJAYI PRANAYAMA

to create UJJAYI BREATH:
- keep LIPS CLOSED
- open the MOUTH INSIDE
- this slightly CONSTRICTS the entry of the THROAT
- Breathe through the NOSE
- your BREATH should make a slight NOISE.

WITH UJJAYI BREATH...

Breathe in through the nose

RETAIN

Breath out through LEFT NOSTRIL

Do ~10 Rounds

LOCK UDDIYANA BANDA during UJJAYI to BREATHE into the DIAPHRAGM

in SAVASANA

Rotate shoulders back, to create more space.

the center of the BREATH is ~2 inches below the NAVEL

to relax the legs:
- in the GAP between outbreath & inbreath, imagine your legs moving together → only in your mind
- on inbreath: relax legs completely

PRANAYAMA is *conscious breathing*

EVERY new BREATH brings new thoughts, EXPECTATIONS & DESIRES
↓
we try to REDUCE the THOUGHTS, EXPECTATIONS & DESIRES
&
JUST ACCEPT our true nature and its beauty

Class poses:

①

② keep back straight, rotate to side

③ open chest — legs active — shoulder on floor; thread one arm underneath to body, other arm over head to floor

④

⑤ 2 rounds of KAPALABATI

⑦ knees from side to side, legs don't touch the floor

⑧ 60 45 30 15

⑨

⑩

⑪ extend left leg to left side on the floor

⑫ activate inner thighs, pull in. leg on wall

⑬ rotate hip first OUT, then IN

⑭ try to get elbow on the floor; forward fold from wide stance

⑮ legs vertical, spread wide, feet active, then lift head.

⑯ lie down, one leg vertical, try to drop it to floor on opposite side, bring it up to your head

⑰

⑱ WARRIOR I

⑲ extended side angle

⑳

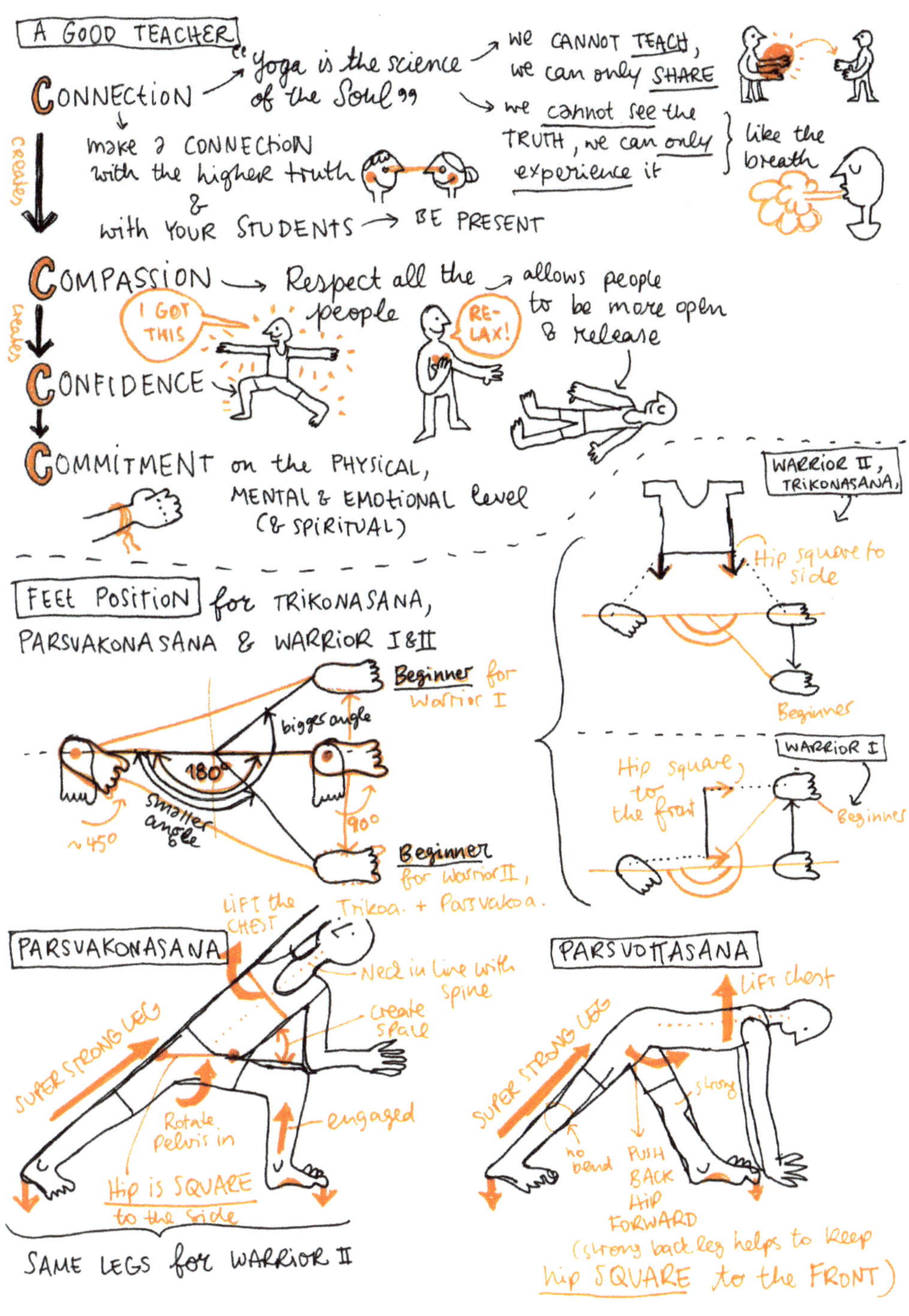

A GOOD TEACHER
CONNECTION
"Yoga is the science of the Soul"
we CANNOT TEACH, we can only SHARE
we cannot see the TRUTH, we can only experience it
like the breath
make a CONNECTION with the higher truth & with YOUR STUDENTS
BE PRESENT
creates
COMPASSION
Respect all the people
allows people to be more open & release
I GOT THIS
RE-LAX!
creates
CONFIDENCE
COMMITMENT on the PHYSICAL, MENTAL & EMOTIONAL level (& SPIRITUAL)
WARRIOR II, TRIKONASANA
Hip square to side
Beginner
FEET POSITION for TRIKONASANA, PARSVAKONASANA & WARRIOR I & II
Beginner for Warrior I
bigger angle
180°
smaller angle
~45°
90°
Beginner for Warrior II, Trikoa. + Parsvakoa.
Hip square to the front
WARRIOR I
Beginner
PARSVAKONASANA
LIFT the CHEST
Neck in line with spine
create space
SUPER STRONG LEG
Rotate pelvis in
engaged
Hip is SQUARE to the Side
SAME LEGS for WARRIOR II
PARSVOTTASANA
lift chest
SUPER STRONG LEG
strong
no bend
PUSH BACK HIP FORWARD
(strong back leg helps to keep hip SQUARE to the FRONT)

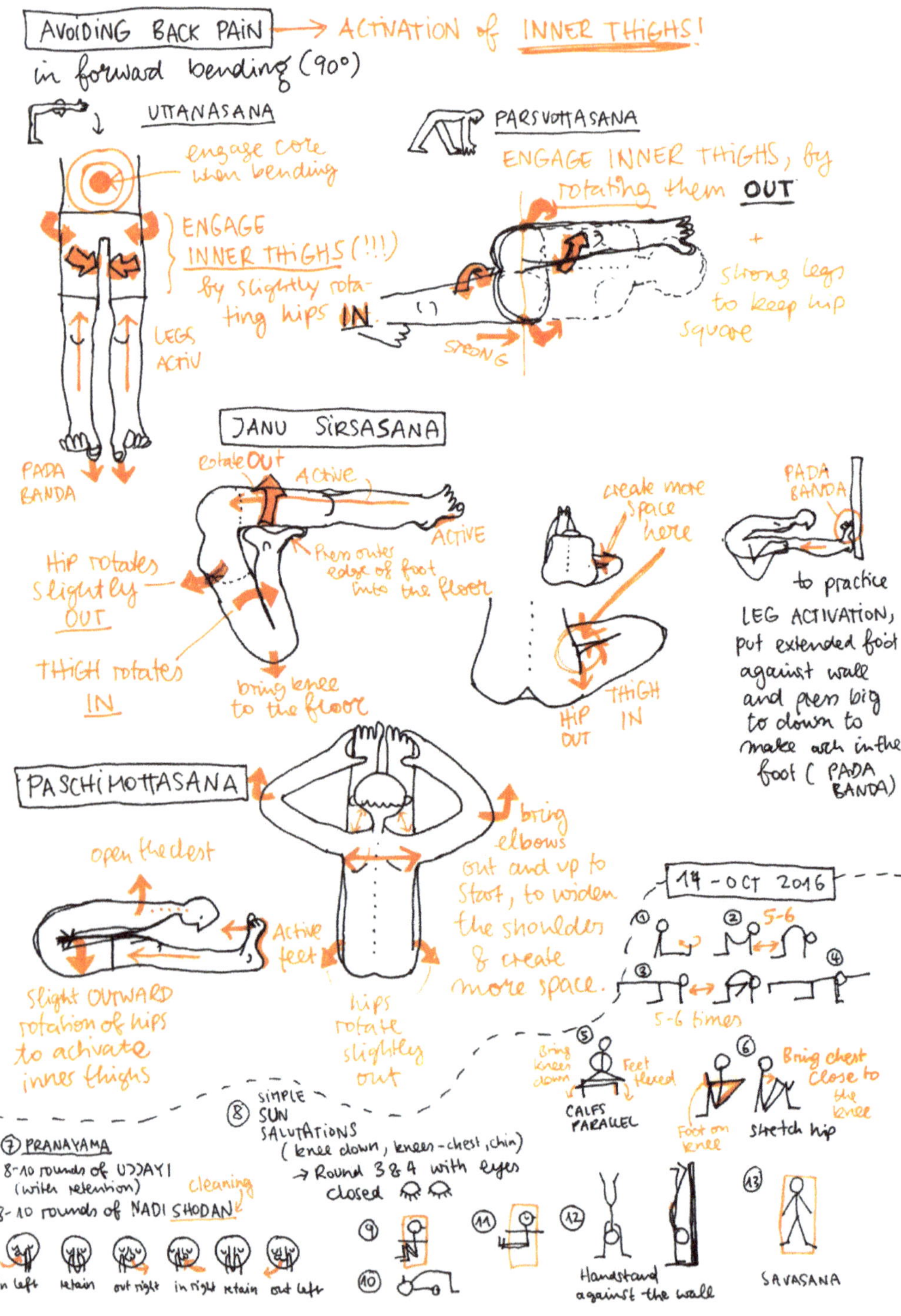

AVOIDING BACK PAIN → ACTIVATION of INNER THIGHS!
in forward bending (90°)

UTTANASANA
engage core when bending
ENGAGE INNER THIGHS (!!!) by slightly rotating hips IN
LEGS ACTIV
PADA BANDA

PARSVOTTASANA
ENGAGE INNER THIGHS, by rotating them OUT
+
strong legs to keep hip square
STRONG

JANU SIRSASANA
rotate OUT
Active
ACTIVE
Press outer edge of foot into the floor
Hip rotates slightly OUT
THIGH rotates IN
bring knee to the floor
create more space here
HIP OUT
THIGH IN
PADA BANDA
to practice LEG ACTIVATION, put extended foot against wall and press big to down to make arch in the foot (PADA BANDA)

PASCHIMOTTASANA
open the chest
Active feet
slight OUTWARD rotation of hips to activate inner thighs
bring elbows out and up to start, to widen the shoulders & create more space.
hips rotate slightly out

14 - OCT 2016
1   2 5-6   4
3   5-6 times
5 Bring knees down   Feet flexed
CALFS PARALLEL
6 Bring chest close to the knee
Foot on knee
stretch hip

⑦ PRANAYAMA
8-10 rounds of UJJAYI (with retention)
8-10 rounds of NADI SHODAN   cleaning
in left   retain   out right   in right   retain   out left

⑧ SIMPLE SUN SALUTATIONS (knee down, knees-chest, chin)
→ Round 3 & 4 with eyes closed

⑨ ⑩ ⑪ ⑫ Handstand against the wall ⑬ SAVASANA

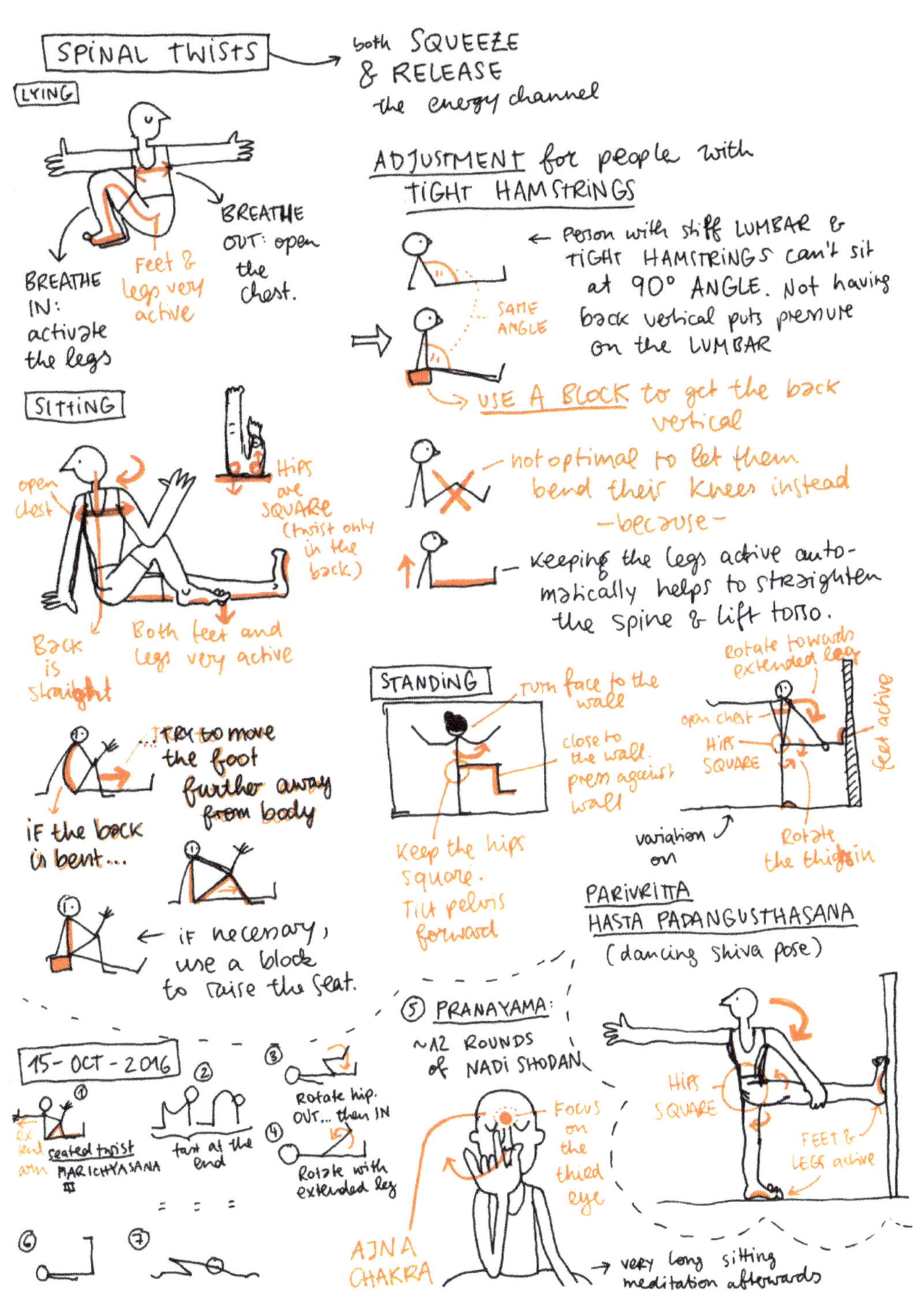

SPINAL TWISTS
both SQUEEZE & RELEASE the energy channel

LYING
BREATHE IN: activate the legs
Feet & legs very active
BREATHE OUT: open the chest.

ADJUSTMENT for people with TIGHT HAMSTRINGS
← Person with stiff LUMBAR & TIGHT HAMSTRINGS can't sit at 90° ANGLE. Not having back vertical puts pressure on the LUMBAR
SAME ANGLE
→ USE A BLOCK to get the back vertical
not optimal to let them bend their knees instead
— because —
keeping the legs active automatically helps to straighten the spine & lift torso.

SITTING
open chest
Hips are SQUARE (twist only in the back)
Back is straight
Both feet and legs very active
Try to move the foot further away from body
if the back is bent...
← if necessary, use a block to raise the seat.

STANDING
turn face to the wall
close to the wall. press against wall
Keep the hips square. Tilt pelvis forward
rotate towards extended leg
open chest
HIPS SQUARE
feet active
variation on
Rotate the thigh in

PARIVRITTA HASTA PADANGUSTHASANA
(dancing shiva pose)
HIPS SQUARE
FEET & LEGS active

15 - OCT - 2016
① ex ten arm seated twist MARICHYASANA III
②
③ Rotate hip. OUT... then IN
tart at the end
④ Rotate with extended leg
⑥ ⑦

⑤ PRANAYAMA:
~12 ROUNDS of NADI SHODAN
Focus on the third eye
AJNA CHAKRA
→ very long sitting meditation afterwards

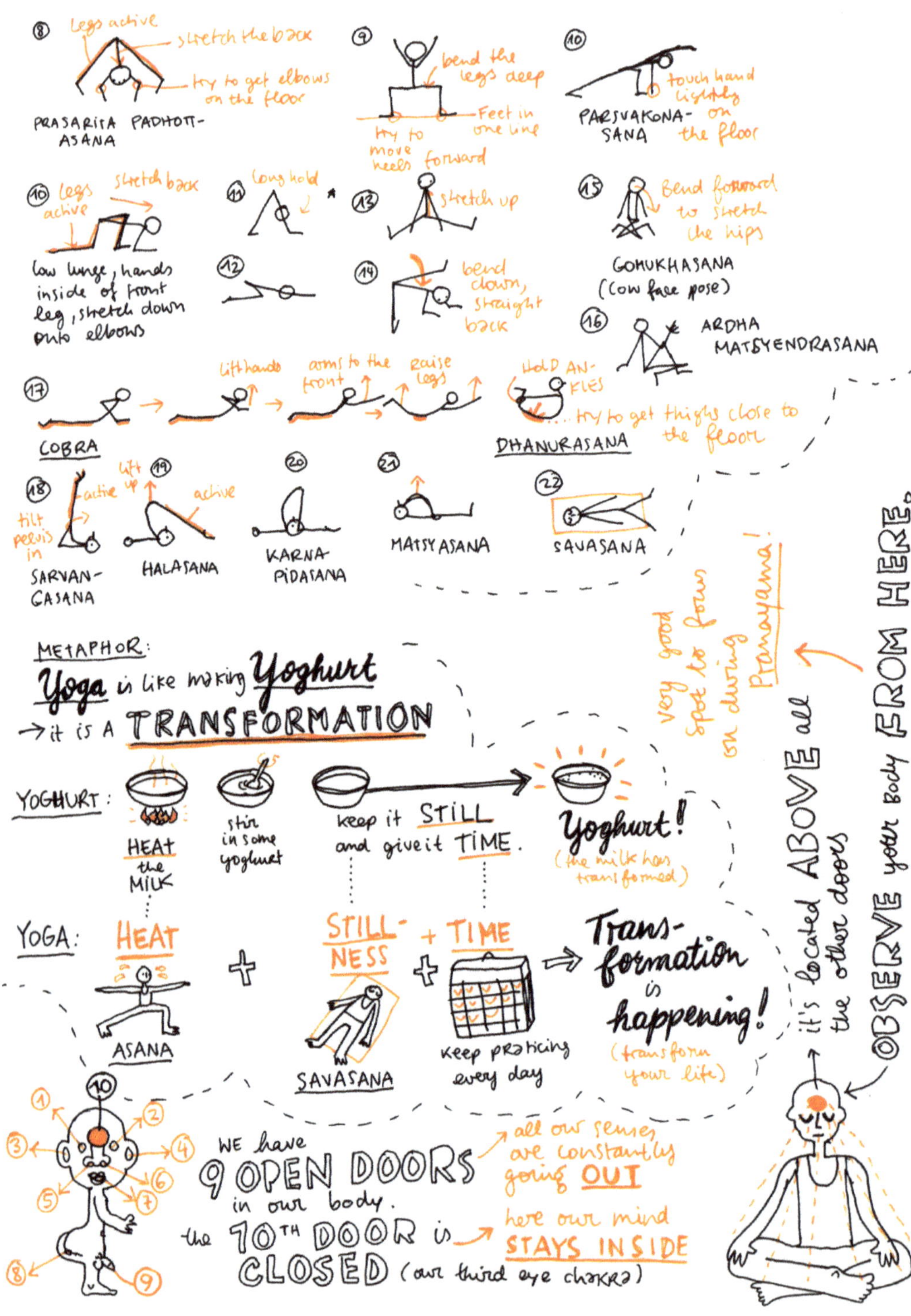

8 Legs active — stretch the back — try to get elbows on the floor
PRASARITA PADHOTT- ASANA

9 bend the legs deep — Feet in one line — try to move heels forward

10 touch hand lightly on the floor
PARSVAKONA- SANA

10 legs active — stretch back
low lunge, hands inside of front leg, stretch down onto elbows

11 Long hold *

13 stretch up

15 Bend forward to stretch the hips
GOMUKHASANA (cow face pose)

12

14 bend down, straight back

16 ARDHA MATSYENDRASANA

17 lift hands — arms to the front — raise legs
COBRA

Hold AN-KLES ... try to get thighs close to the floor
DHANURASANA

18 tilt pelvis in — active — lift up
SARVAN- GASANA

19 active
HALASANA

20 KARNA PIDASANA

21 MATSYASANA

22 SAVASANA

Very good spot to focus on during Pranayama!

ABOVE all the other doors — it's located
OBSERVE your body FROM HERE.

METAPHOR:
Yoga is like making Yoghurt
→ it is a TRANSFORMATION

YOGHURT:
HEAT the MILK
stir in some yoghurt
keep it STILL and give it TIME.
Yoghurt! (the milk has transformed)

YOGA:
HEAT + STILL-NESS + TIME → Transformation is happening! (transform your life)
ASANA
SAVASANA
keep practicing every day

10
1 2 3 4 5 6 7 8 9
WE have 9 OPEN DOORS in our body.
the 10TH DOOR is CLOSED (our third eye chakra)
all our senses are constantly going OUT
here our mind STAYS INSIDE

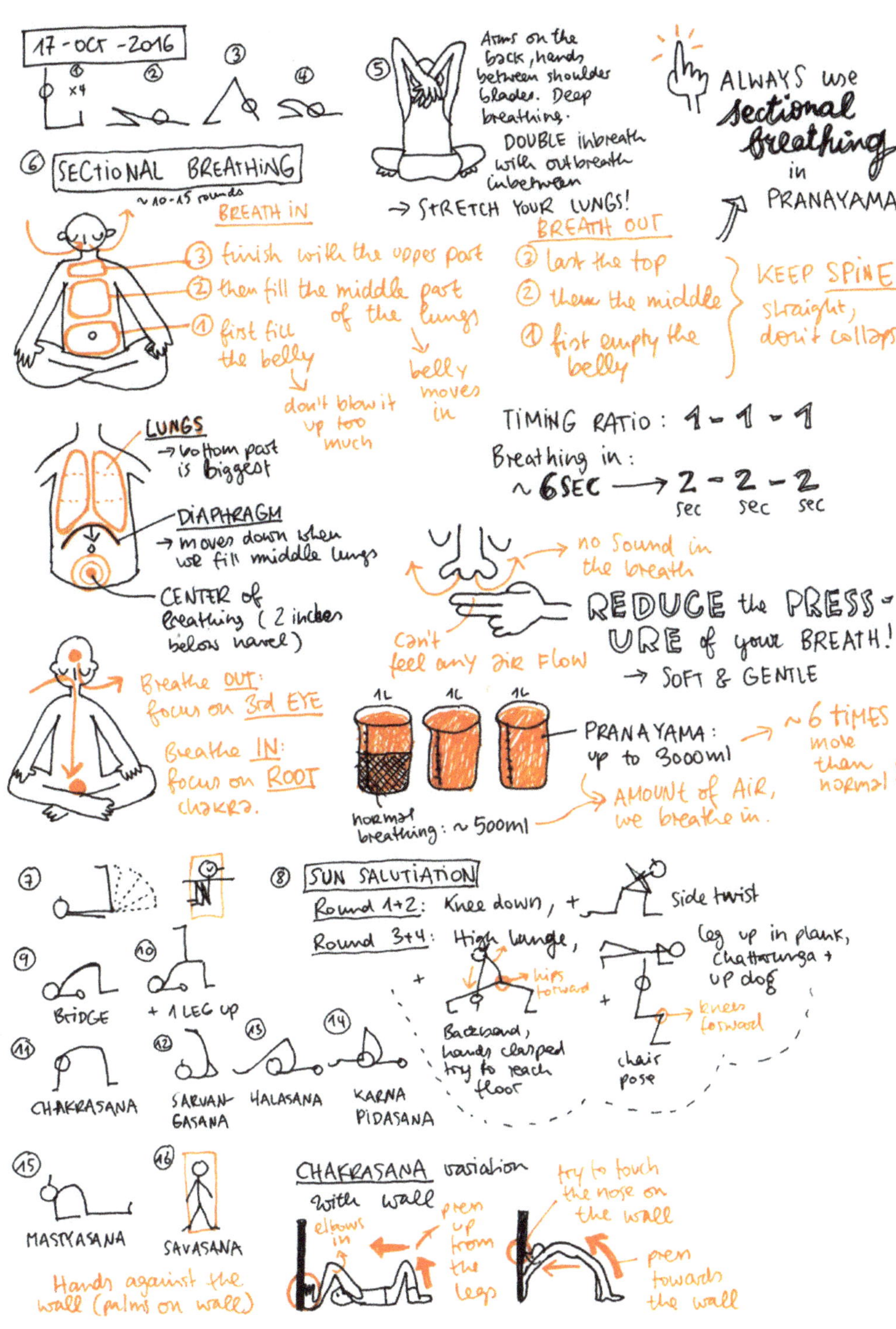

17 - OCT - 2016
x4
⑥ SECTIONAL BREATHING
~ 10-15 rounds
BREATH IN
③ finish with the upper part
② then fill the middle part of the lungs
① first fill the belly
don't blow it up too much
⑤ Arms on the back, hands between shoulder blades. Deep breathing.
DOUBLE inbreath with outbreath inbetween
→ STRETCH YOUR LUNGS!
BREATH OUT
③ last the top
② then the middle
① first empty the belly
belly moves in
ALWAYS use sectional breathing in PRANAYAMA
KEEP SPINE straight; don't collapse
LUNGS
→ bottom part is biggest
DIAPHRAGM
→ moves down when we fill middle lungs
CENTER of breathing (2 inches below navel)
TIMING RATIO: 1 - 1 - 1
Breathing in: ~ 6 SEC → 2 - 2 - 2
sec sec sec
no sound in the breath
can't feel any air flow
REDUCE the PRESSURE of your BREATH!
→ SOFT & GENTLE
Breathe OUT: focus on 3rd EYE
Breathe IN: focus on ROOT chakra.
1L 1L 1L
normal breathing: ~ 500ml
PRANAYAMA: up to 3000ml
→ ~ 6 TIMES more than normal!
AMOUNT of AIR, we breathe in.
⑦
⑧ SUN SALUTIATION
Round 1+2: Knee down, + Side twist
Round 3+4: High lunge,
hips forward
Backbend, hands clasped try to reach floor
Leg up in plank, Chaturanga + up dog
knees forward
chair pose
⑨ ⑩ + 1 LEG UP
BRIDGE
⑪ CHAKRASANA
⑫ SARVAN GASANA
⑬ HALASANA
⑭ KARNA PIDASANA
⑮ MASTYASANA
⑯ SAVASANA
Hands against the wall (palms on wall)
CHAKRASANA variation with wall
press up from the legs
elbows in
try to touch the nose on the wall
press towards the wall

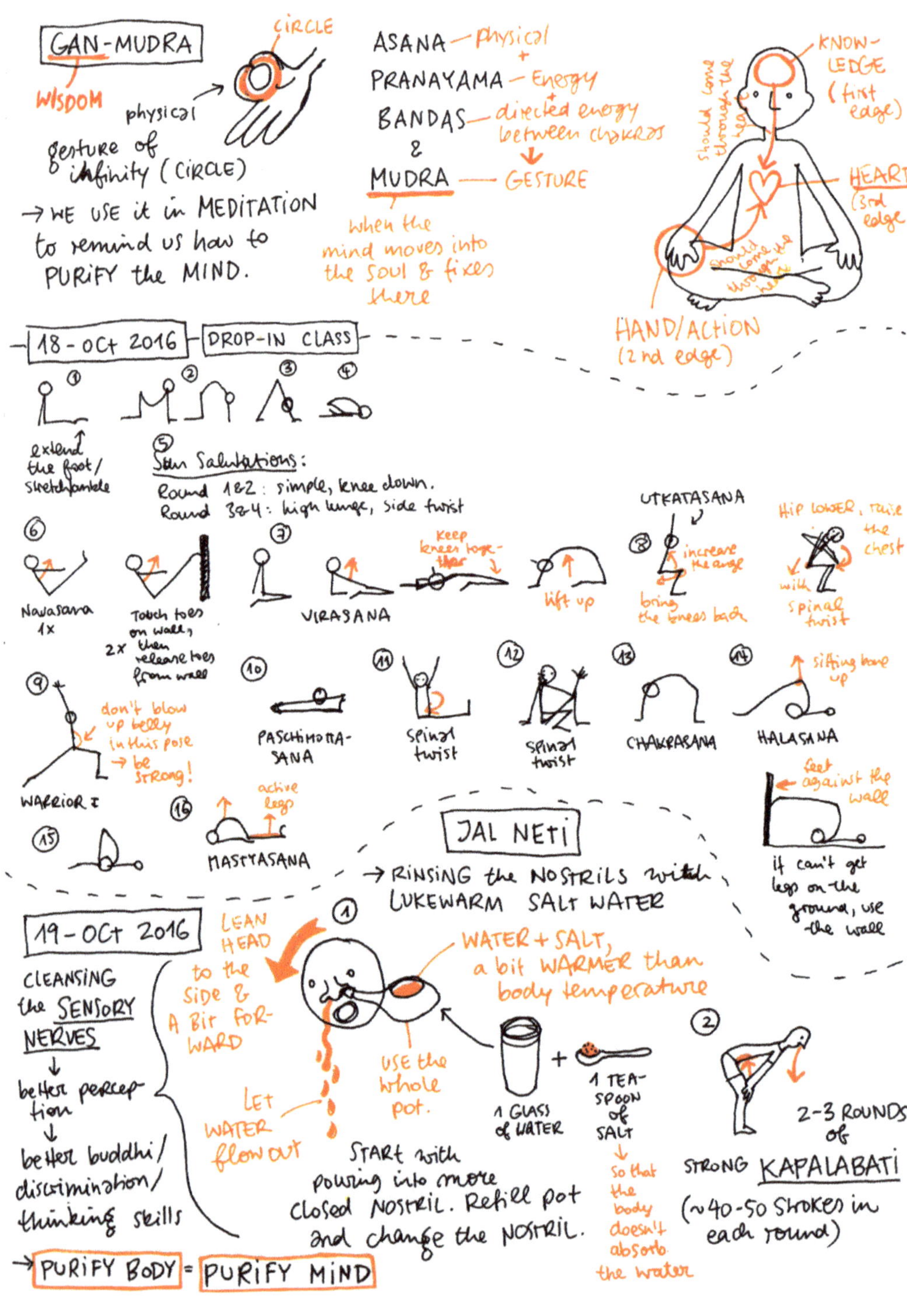

GAN-MUDRA
CIRCLE
WISDOM
physical gesture of infinity (CIRCLE)
→ WE USE it in MEDITATION to remind us how to PURIFY the MIND.

ASANA — physical
+
PRANAYAMA — Energy
+
BANDAS — directed energy between chakras
&
MUDRA — GESTURE
when the mind moves into the soul & fixes there

KNOW-LEDGE (first edge)
should come through the head
HEART (3rd edge)
should come through the heart
HAND/ACTION (2nd edge)

18 - OCT 2016   DROP-IN CLASS
① ② ③ ④
extend the foot / stretch ankle
⑤ Sun Salutations:
Round 1&2: simple, knee down.
Round 3&4: high lunge, side twist

⑥ Navasana 1x
Touch toes on wall, then release toes from wall 2x
⑦ VIRASANA
keep knees together
lift up
UTKATASANA
⑧ increase the angle
bring the knees back
Hip LOWER, raise the chest
with spinal twist

⑨ WARRIOR I
don't blow up belly in this pose → be strong!
⑩ PASCHIMOTTA-SANA
⑪ Spinal twist
⑫ Spinal twist
⑬ CHAKRASANA
⑭ HALASANA
sitting bone up
feet against the wall
if can't get legs on the ground, use the wall

⑮ ⑯ MATSYASANA
active legs

JAL NETI
→ RINSING the NOSTRILS with LUKEWARM SALT WATER

19 - OCT 2016
CLEANSING the SENSORY NERVES
↓
better perception
↓
better buddhi / discrimination / thinking skills
→ PURIFY BODY = PURIFY MIND

① LEAN HEAD to the side & A BIT FORWARD
WATER + SALT, a bit WARMER than body temperature
USE the whole pot.
LET WATER flow out
START with pouring into more closed NOSTRIL. Refill pot and change the NOSTRIL.
1 GLASS of WATER
+
1 TEA-SPOON of SALT
↓
so that the body doesn't absorb the water

② 2-3 ROUNDS of STRONG KAPALABATI
(~40-50 strokes in each round)

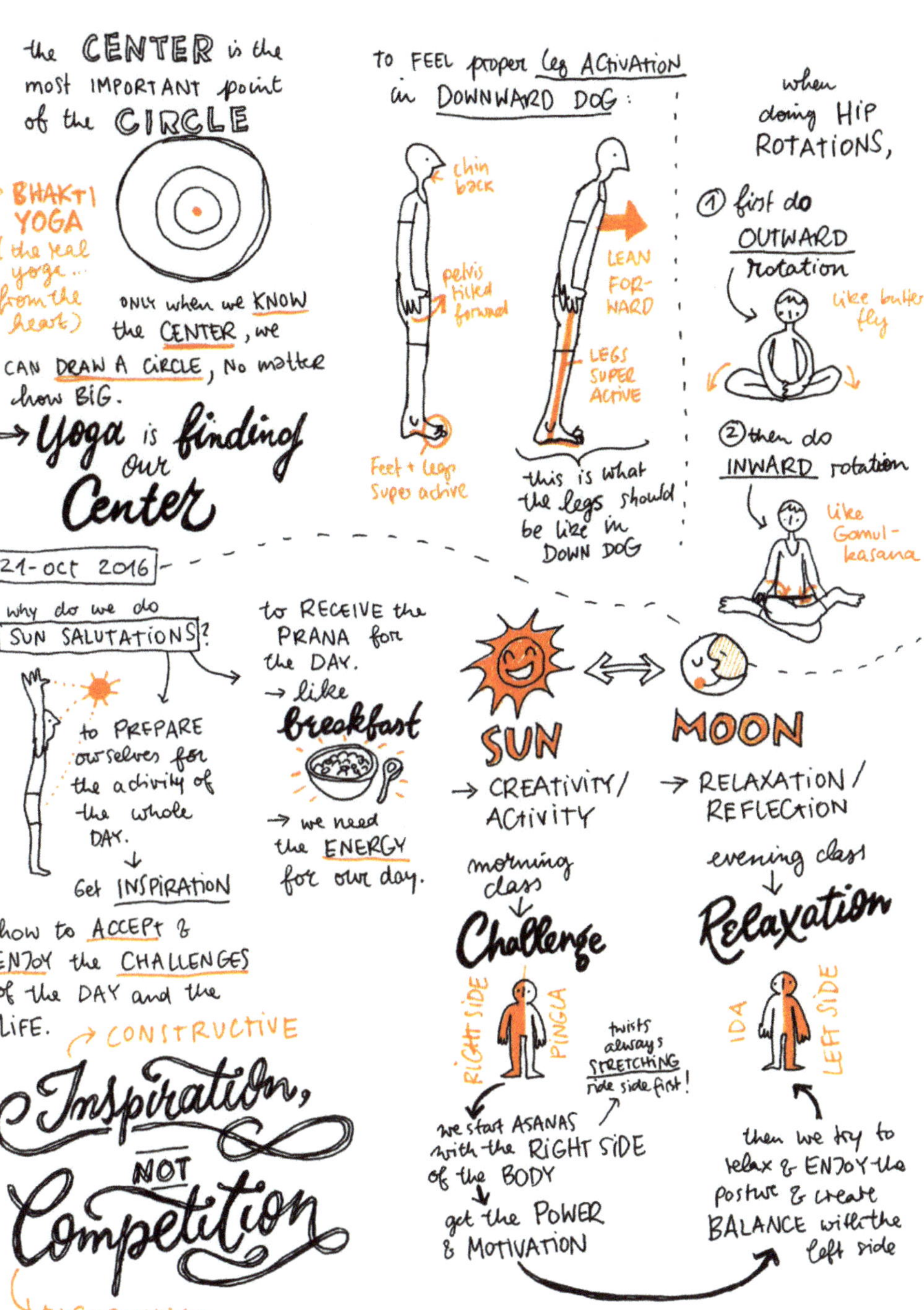

the CENTER is the most IMPORTANT point of the CIRCLE

→ BHAKTI YOGA (the real yoga... from the heart)

ONLY when we KNOW the CENTER, we CAN DRAW A CIRCLE, no matter how BIG.

→ Yoga is finding our Center

- 21-oct 2016 -

why do we do SUN SALUTATIONS?

to PREPARE ourselves for the activity of the whole DAY.
↓
Get INSPIRATION

how to ACCEPT & ENJOY the CHALLENGES of the DAY and the LIFE.

→ CONSTRUCTIVE

Inspiration, NOT Competition

↳ DESTRUCTIVE

TO FEEL proper Leg ACTIVATION in DOWNWARD DOG:

chin back

pelvis tilted forward

Feet + legs super active

LEAN FORWARD

LEGS SUPER ACTIVE

this is what the legs should be like in DOWN DOG

to RECEIVE the PRANA for the DAY.
→ like breakfast
→ we need the ENERGY for our day.

when doing HIP ROTATIONS,

① first do OUTWARD rotation
like butter-fly

② then do INWARD rotation
like Gomul-kasana

SUN ⟷ MOON

SUN → CREATIVITY / ACTIVITY

morning class
↓
Challenge

RIGHT SIDE   PINGLA

twists always STRETCHING ride side first!

we start ASANAS with the RIGHT SIDE of the BODY
↓
get the POWER & MOTIVATION

MOON → RELAXATION / REFLECTION

evening class
↓
Relaxation

IDA   LEFT SIDE

then we try to relax & ENJOY the posture & create BALANCE with the left side

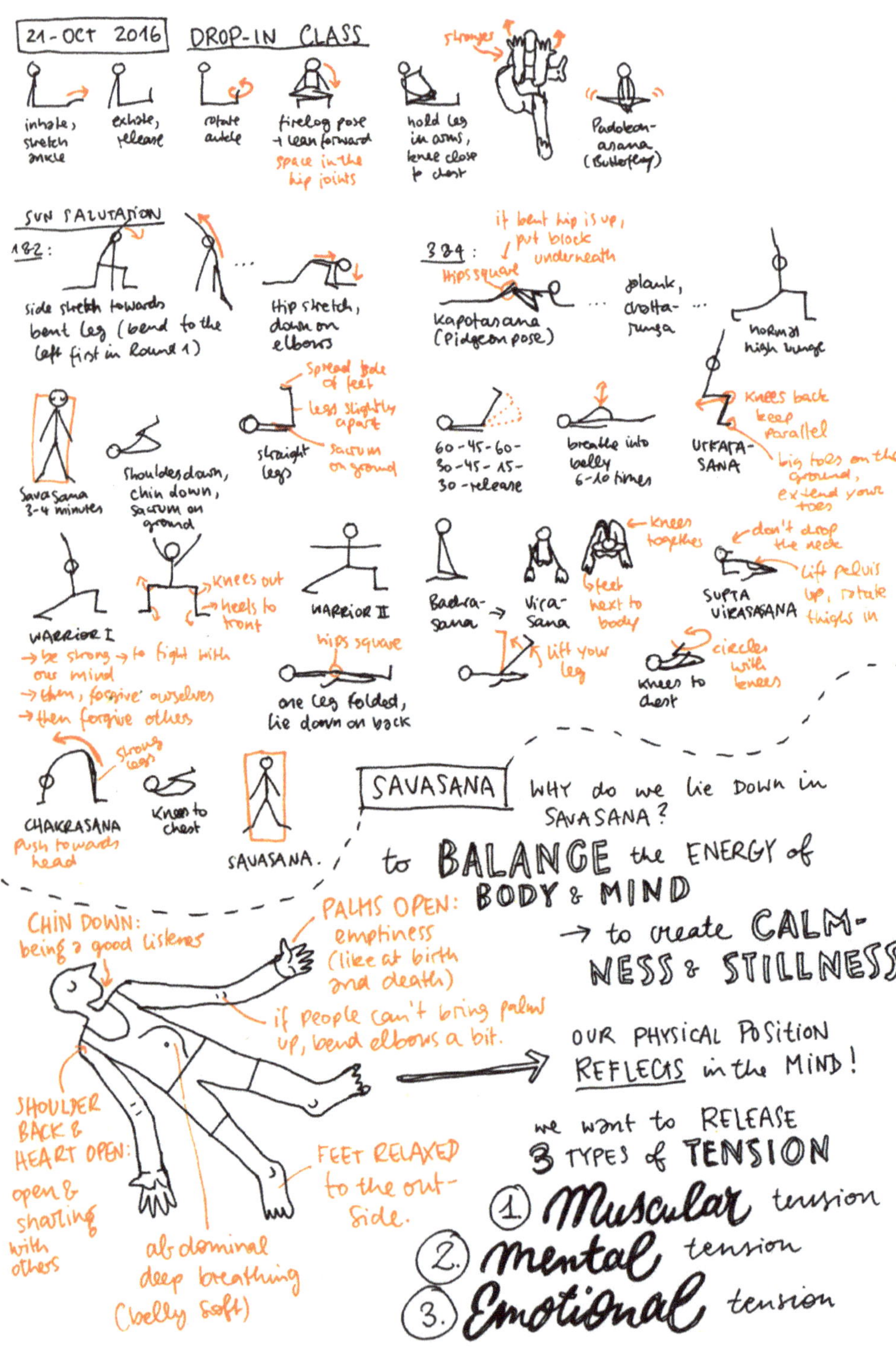

21-OCT 2016   DROP-IN CLASS

inhale, stretch ankle
exhale, release
rotate ankle
firelog pose + lean forward
space in the hip joints
hold leg in arms, knee close to chest
stronger
Padotanasana (Butterfly)

SUN SALUTATION
1 & 2:
side stretch towards bent leg (bend to the left first in Round 1)
Hip stretch, down on elbows

3 & 4:
if bent hip is up, put block underneath
hips square
Kapotasana (Pidgeon pose)
plank, chaturunga
normal high lunge

Savasana 3-4 minutes
shoulders down, chin down, sacrum on ground
spread sole of feet
legs slightly apart
sacrum on ground
straight legs
60-45-60-30-45-15-30-release
breathe into belly 6-10 times
UTKATASANA
knees back keep parallel
big toes on the ground, extend your toes

WARRIOR I
→ be strong → to fight with our mind
→ then, forgive ourselves
→ then forgive others
knees out
heels to front
WARRIOR II
hips square
one leg folded, lie down on back
Badrasana
Virasana
knees together
feet next to body
SUPTA VIRASASANA
don't drop the neck
lift pelvis up, rotate thighs in
lift your leg
knees to chest
circles with knees

CHAKRASANA
push towards head
strong legs
knees to chest
SAVASANA.

SAVASANA   WHY do we lie DOWN in SAVASANA?
to BALANCE the ENERGY of BODY & MIND
→ to create CALM-NESS & STILLNESS

OUR PHYSICAL POSITION REFLECTS in the MIND!

we want to RELEASE 3 TYPES of TENSION
① Muscular tension
②. mental tension
③. Emotional tension

CHIN DOWN: being a good listener
PALMS OPEN: emptiness (like at birth and death)
if people can't bring palms up, bend elbows a bit.
SHOULDER BACK & HEART OPEN: open & sharing with others
abdominal deep breathing (belly soft)
FEET RELAXED to the out-side.

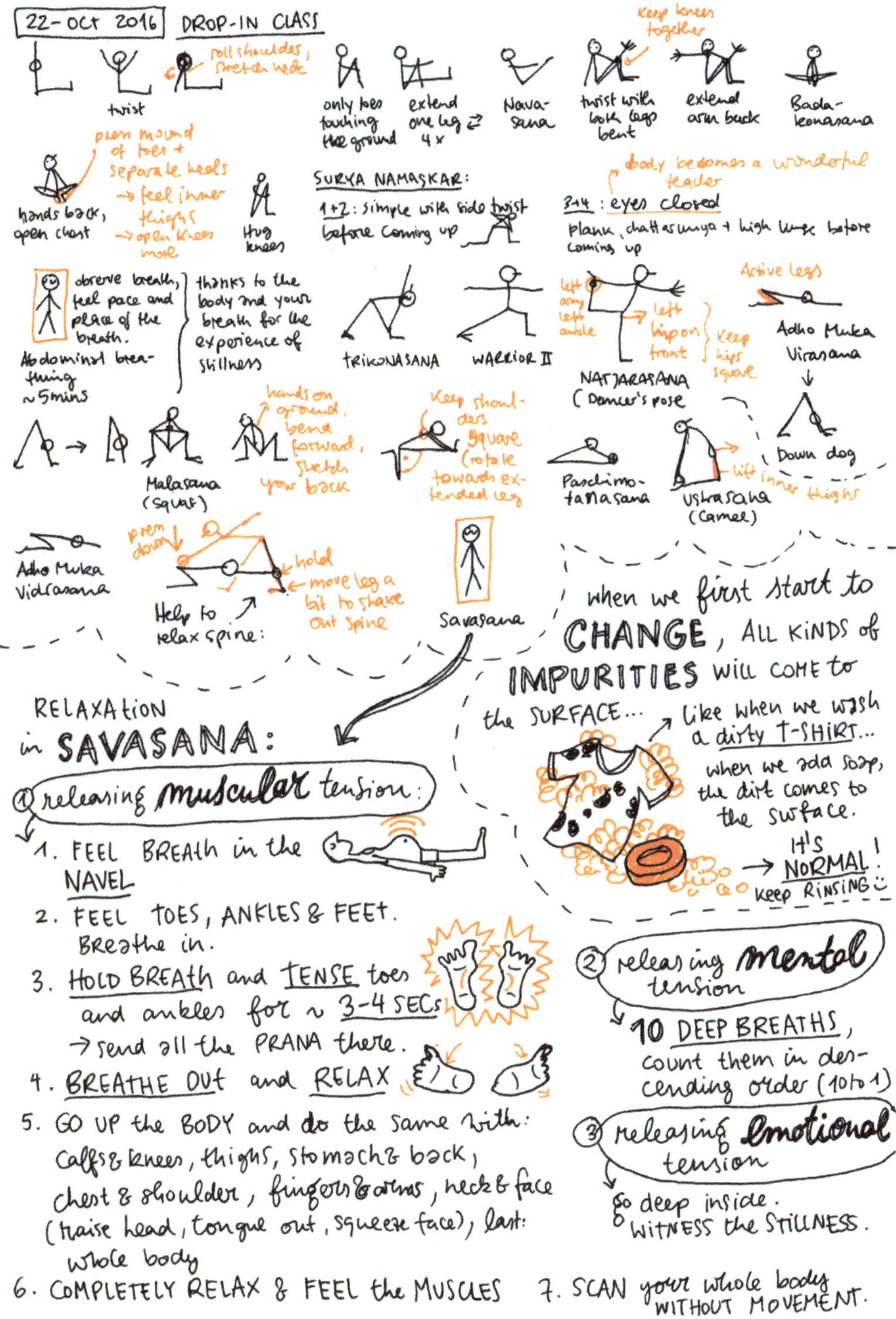

22-OCT 2016 DROP-IN CLASS
twist
roll shoulders, stretch neck
only toes touching the ground
extend one leg 4x
Nava-sana
Keep knees together
twist with both legs bent
extend arm back
Bada-konasana
hands back, open chest
press mound of toes + separate heels
→ feel inner thighs
→ open knees more
Hug knees
SURYA NAMASKAR:
1+2: simple with side twist before coming up
body becomes a wonderful teacher
3+4: eyes closed
plank, chattarunga + high lunge before coming up
observe breath, feel pace and place of the breath.
Abdominal breathing ~5mins
thanks to the body and your breath for the experience of stillness
TRIKONASANA
WARRIOR II
left arm left ankle
left hip on front
Keep hips square
Active legs
Adho Muka Virasana
NATJARASANA (Dancer's pose)
hands on ground, bend forward, stretch your back
Malasana (squat)
Keep shoulders square (rotate towards extended leg
Paschimo-tanasana
Ustrasana (Camel)
lift inner thighs
Down dog
Adho Muka Vidrasana
press down
Help to relax spine:
hold
move leg a bit to shake out spine
Savasana
when we first start to CHANGE, ALL KINDS of IMPURITIES WILL COME to the SURFACE...
like when we wash a dirty T-SHIRT...
when we add soap, the dirt comes to the surface.
It's NORMAL!
keep RINSING
RELAXATION in SAVASANA:
① releasing muscular tension:
1. FEEL BREATH in the NAVEL
2. FEEL TOES, ANKLES & FEET. Breathe in.
3. HOLD BREATH and TENSE toes and ankles for ~ 3-4 SECs
→ send all the PRANA there.
4. BREATHE OUT and RELAX
5. GO UP the BODY and do the same with: calfs & knees, thighs, stomach & back, chest & shoulder, fingers & arms, neck & face (raise head, tongue out, squeeze face), last: whole body
6. COMPLETELY RELAX & FEEL the MUSCLES
② releasing mental tension
10 DEEP BREATHS, count them in descending order (10 to 1)
③ releasing emotional tension
go deep inside. WITNESS the STILLNESS.
7. SCAN your whole body WITHOUT MOVEMENT.

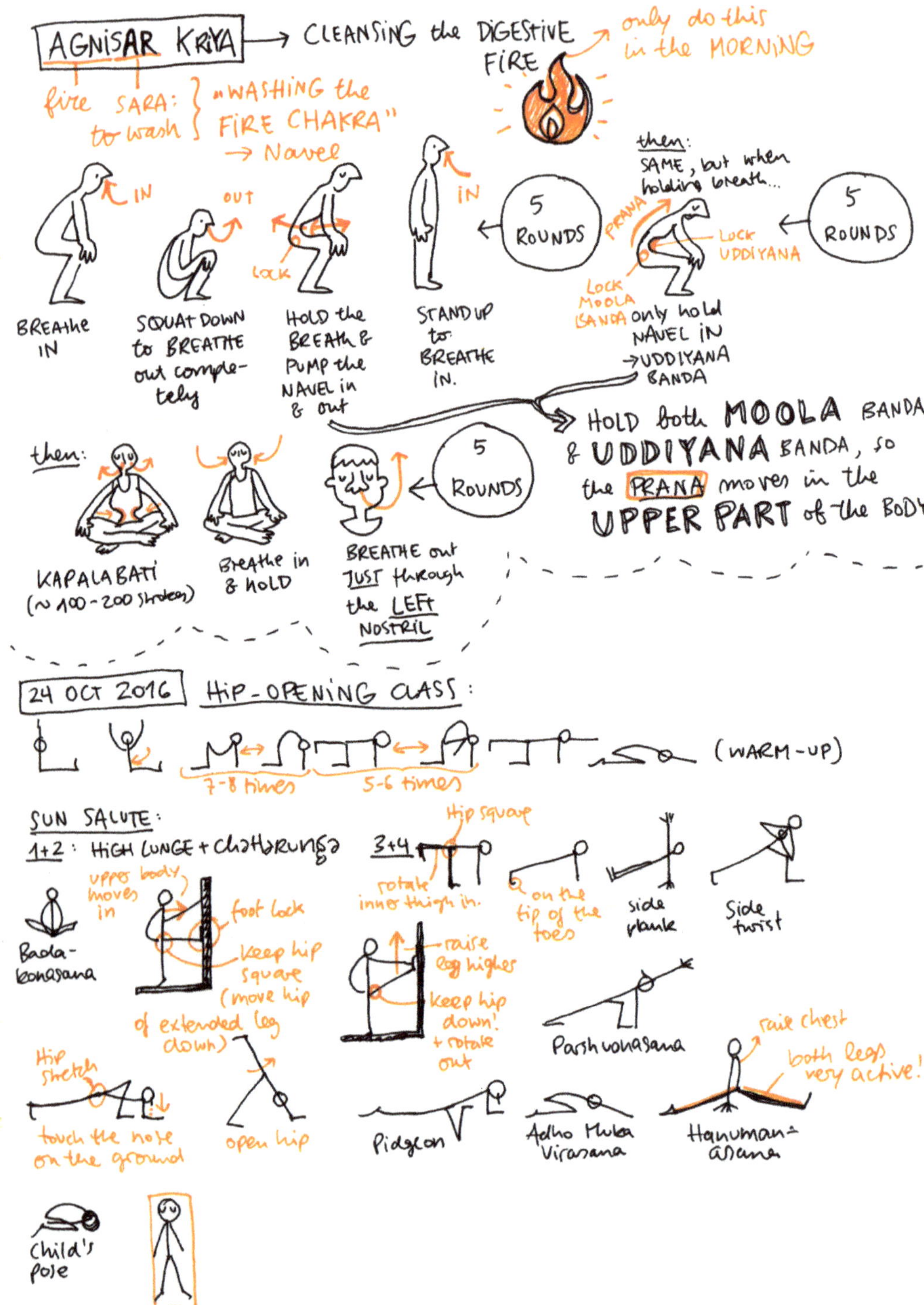

AGNISAR KRIYA → CLEANSING the DIGESTIVE FIRE → only do this in the MORNING

fire SARA: to wash } "WASHING the FIRE CHAKRA" → Navel

IN
out
lock
Lock

BREATHE IN

SQUAT DOWN to BREATHE out comple-tely

HOLD the BREATH & PUMP the NAVEL in & out

STAND UP to BREATHE IN.

IN

5 ROUNDS

then: SAME, but when holding breath...

PRANA
LOCK MOOLA BANDA
LOCK UDDIYANA
only hold NAVEL IN → UDDIYANA BANDA

5 ROUNDS

HOLD both MOOLA BANDA & UDDIYANA BANDA, so the PRANA moves in the UPPER PART of the BODY.

then:
KAPALABATI (~ 100-200 Strokes)

Breathe in & HOLD

BREATHE out JUST through the LEFT NOSTRIL

5 ROUNDS

24 OCT 2016 HIP-OPENING CLASS:
7-8 times   5-6 times   (WARM-UP)

SUN SALUTE:
1+2: HIGH LUNGE + Chaturanga

Hip square
3+4
rotate inner thigh in.

upper body moves in
foot lock
keep hip square (move hip of extended leg down)

Baoda-konasana

raise leg higher
keep hip down! + rotate out

on the tip of the toes

side plank

Side twist

Parshvokasana

raise chest
both legs very active!

Hip stretch
touch the nose on the ground

open hip

Pidgeon

Adho Mukha Virasana

Hanuman-asana

Child's pose

Savasana

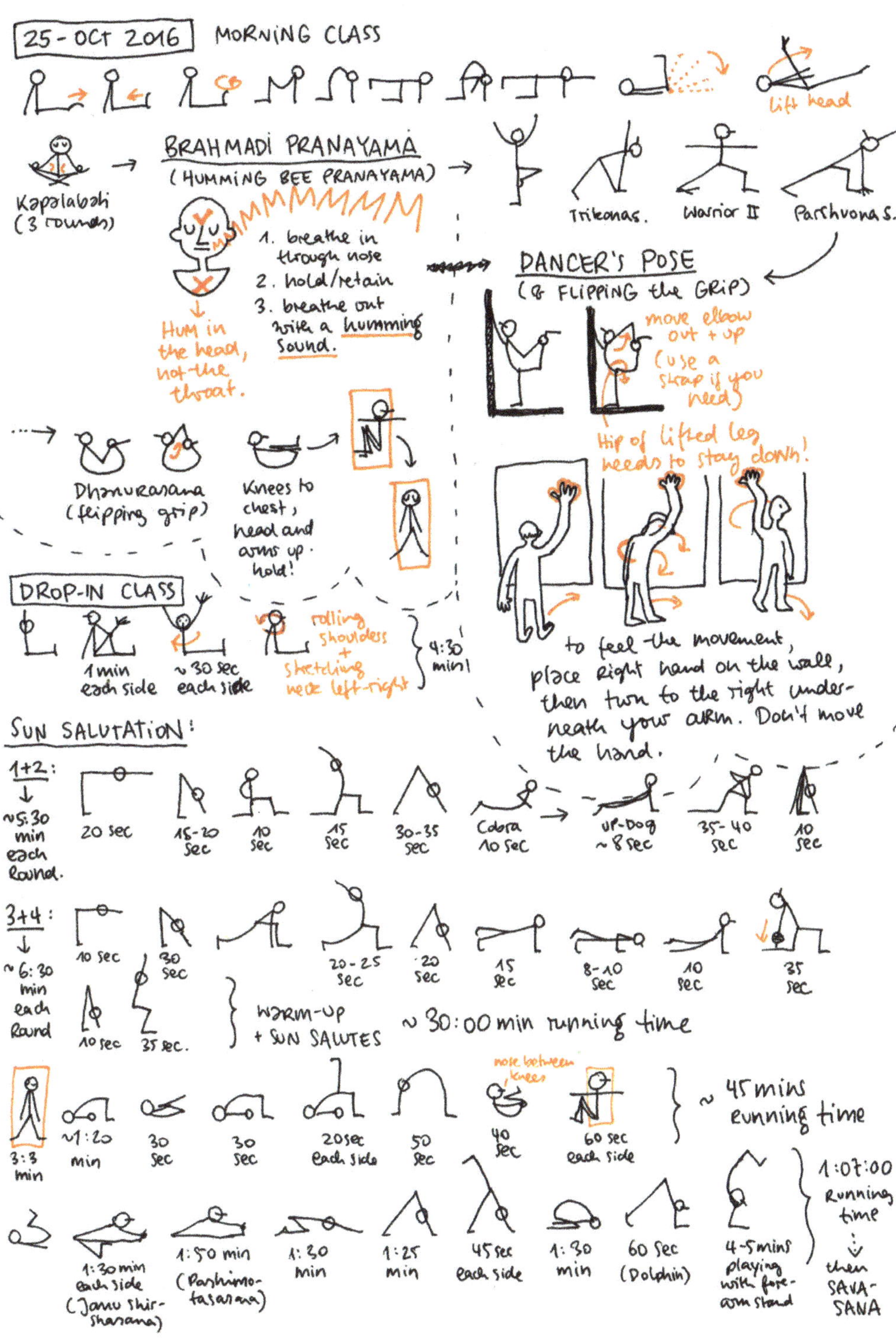

25 - OCT 2016   MORNING CLASS

Kapalabati
(3 rounds)

BRAHMADI PRANAYAMA
(HUMMING BEE PRANAYAMA)

MMMMMMM

1. breathe in through nose
2. hold/retain
3. breathe out with a humming sound.

Hum in the head, not the throat.

Trikonas.   Warrior II   Parshvona S.

lift head

DANCER'S POSE
(& FLIPPING the GRIP)

move elbow out + up
(use a strap if you need)

Hip of lifted leg needs to stay down!

Dhanurasana
(flipping grip)

Knees to chest, head and arms up. hold!

DROP-IN CLASS

1 min each side

~30 sec each side

rolling shoulders + stretching neck left-right

4:30 min!

to feel the movement, place right hand on the wall, then turn to the right underneath your arm. Don't move the hand.

SUN SALUTATION:

1+2:
↓
~5:30 min each round.

20 sec   15-20 sec   10 sec   15 sec   30-35 sec   Cobra 10 sec   up-Dog ~8 sec   35-40 sec   10 sec

3+4:
↓
~6:30 min each Round

10 sec   30 sec   20-25 sec   20 sec   15 sec   8-10 sec   10 sec   35 sec

10 sec   35 sec.

WARM-UP + SUN SALUTES   ~30:00 min running time

nose between knees

~45 mins running time

3:3 min   ~1:20 min   30 sec   30 sec   20 sec each side   50 sec   40 sec   60 sec each side

1:07:00 running time
↓
then SAVASANA

1:30 min each side (Janu Shirshasana)   1:50 min (Parshimotasana)   1:30 min   1:25 min   45 sec each side   1:30 min   60 sec (Dolphin)   4-5 mins playing with forearm stand

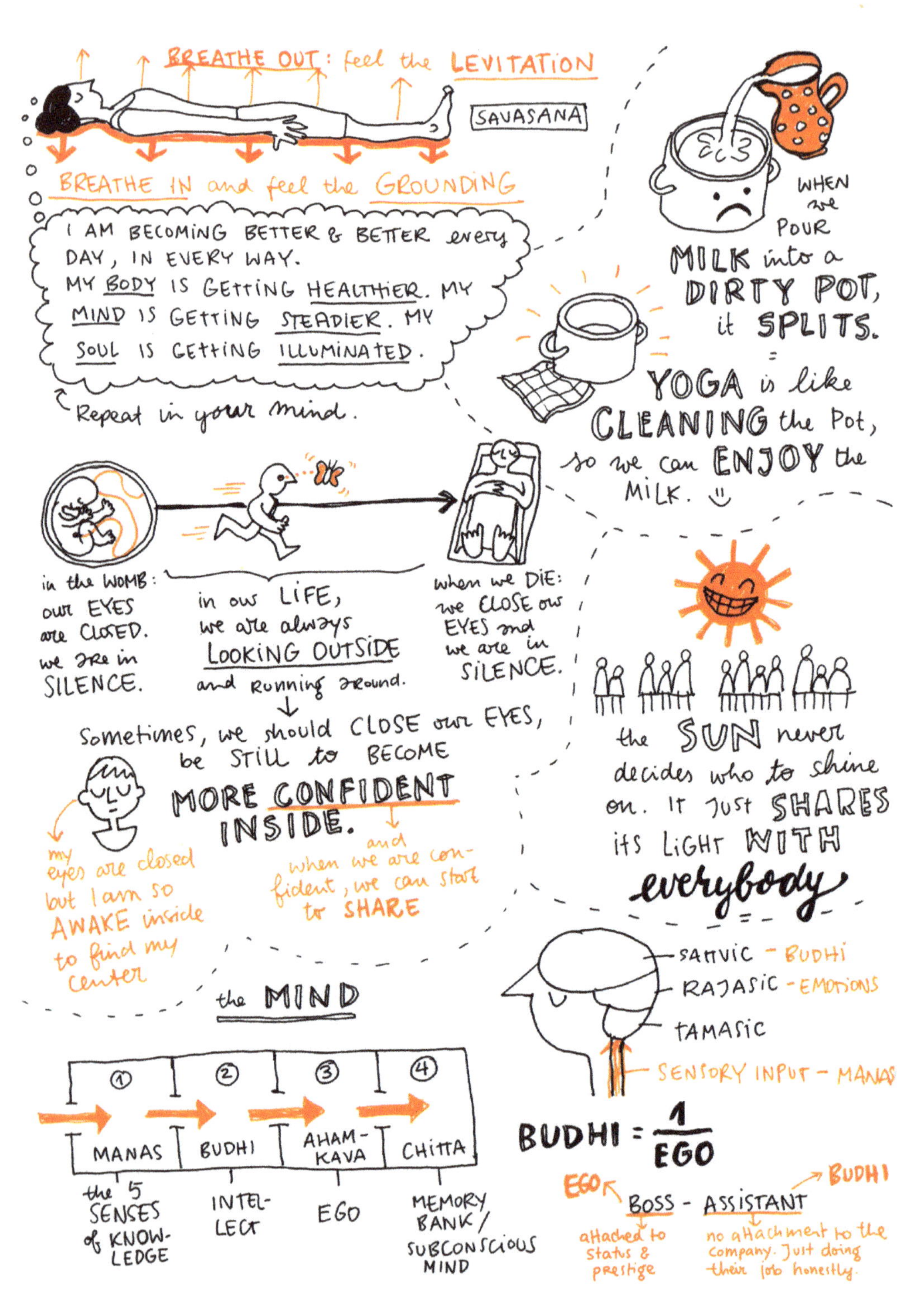

BREATHE OUT: feel the LEVITATION
SAVASANA
BREATHE IN and feel the GROUNDING

I AM BECOMING BETTER & BETTER every DAY, IN EVERY WAY.
MY BODY IS GETTING HEALTHIER. MY MIND IS GETTING STEADIER. MY SOUL IS GETTING ILLUMINATED.
Repeat in your mind.

WHEN we POUR MILK into a DIRTY POT, it SPLITS.
=
YOGA is like CLEANING the Pot, so we can ENJOY the MILK. ☺

in the WOMB: our EYES are CLOSED. we are in SILENCE.
in our LIFE, we are always LOOKING OUTSIDE and running around.
when we DIE: we CLOSE our EYES and we are in SILENCE.

Sometimes, we should CLOSE our EYES, be STILL to BECOME MORE CONFIDENT INSIDE.

my eyes are closed but I am so AWAKE inside to find my center

and when we are confident, we can start to SHARE

the SUN never decides who to shine on. It just SHARES its LIGHT WITH everybody

SATTVIC — BUDHI
RAJASIC — EMOTIONS
TAMASIC
SENSORY INPUT — MANAS

the MIND

① MANAS
② BUDHI
③ AHAM-KAVA
④ CHITTA

the 5 SENSES of KNOWLEDGE
INTELLECT
EGO
MEMORY BANK / SUBCONSCIOUS MIND

BUDHI = 1/EGO

EGO
BUDHI
BOSS - ASSISTANT
attached to status & prestige
no attachment to the company. Just doing their job honestly.

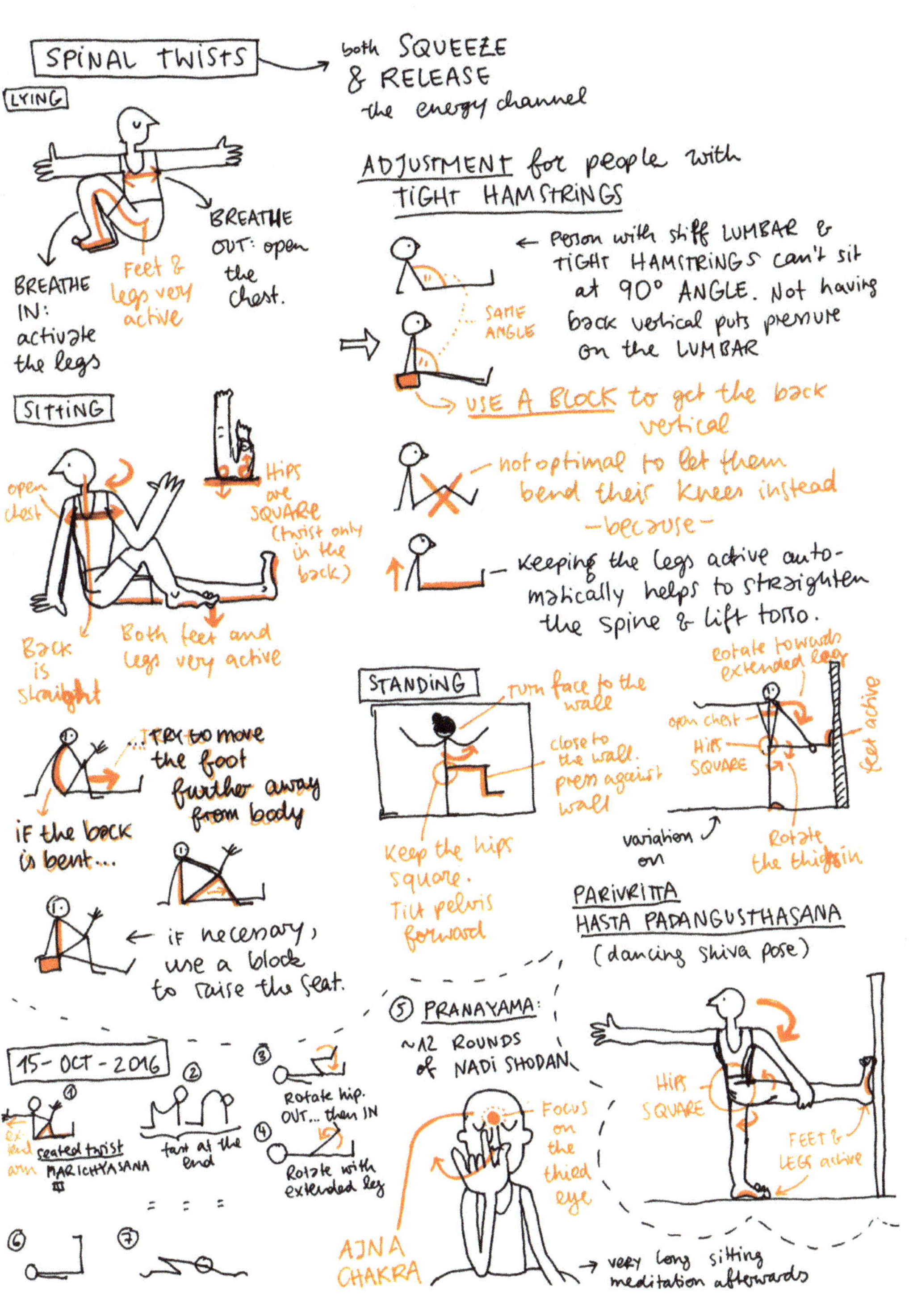

SPINAL TWISTS

both SQUEEZE & RELEASE the energy channel

LYING

BREATHE IN: activate the legs

Feet & legs very active

BREATHE OUT: open the chest.

SITTING

open chest

Back is straight

Both feet and legs very active

Hips are SQUARE (twist only in the back)

...TRY to move the foot further away from body

if the back is bent...

if necessary, use a block to raise the seat.

ADJUSTMENT for people with TIGHT HAMSTRINGS

← Person with stiff LUMBAR & TIGHT HAMSTRINGS can't sit at 90° ANGLE. Not having back vertical puts pressure on the LUMBAR

SAME ANGLE

→ USE A BLOCK to get the back vertical

not optimal to let them bend their knees instead

—because—

keeping the legs active automatically helps to straighten the spine & lift torso.

STANDING

turn face to the wall

close to the wall. press against wall

Keep the hips square. Tilt pelvis forward

open chest
HIPS SQUARE
feet active

rotate towards extended leg

variation on

Rotate the thigh in

PARIVRITTA HASTA PADANGUSTHASANA (dancing shiva pose)

HIPS SQUARE

FEET & LEGS active

15 - OCT - 2016

① extend arm
seated twist
MARICHYASANA III

② fast at the end

③

④ Rotate with extended leg

Rotate hip. OUT... then IN

⑤ PRANAYAMA: ~12 ROUNDS of NADI SHODAN.

Focus on the third eye

AJNA CHAKRA

→ very long sitting meditation afterwards

⑥

⑦

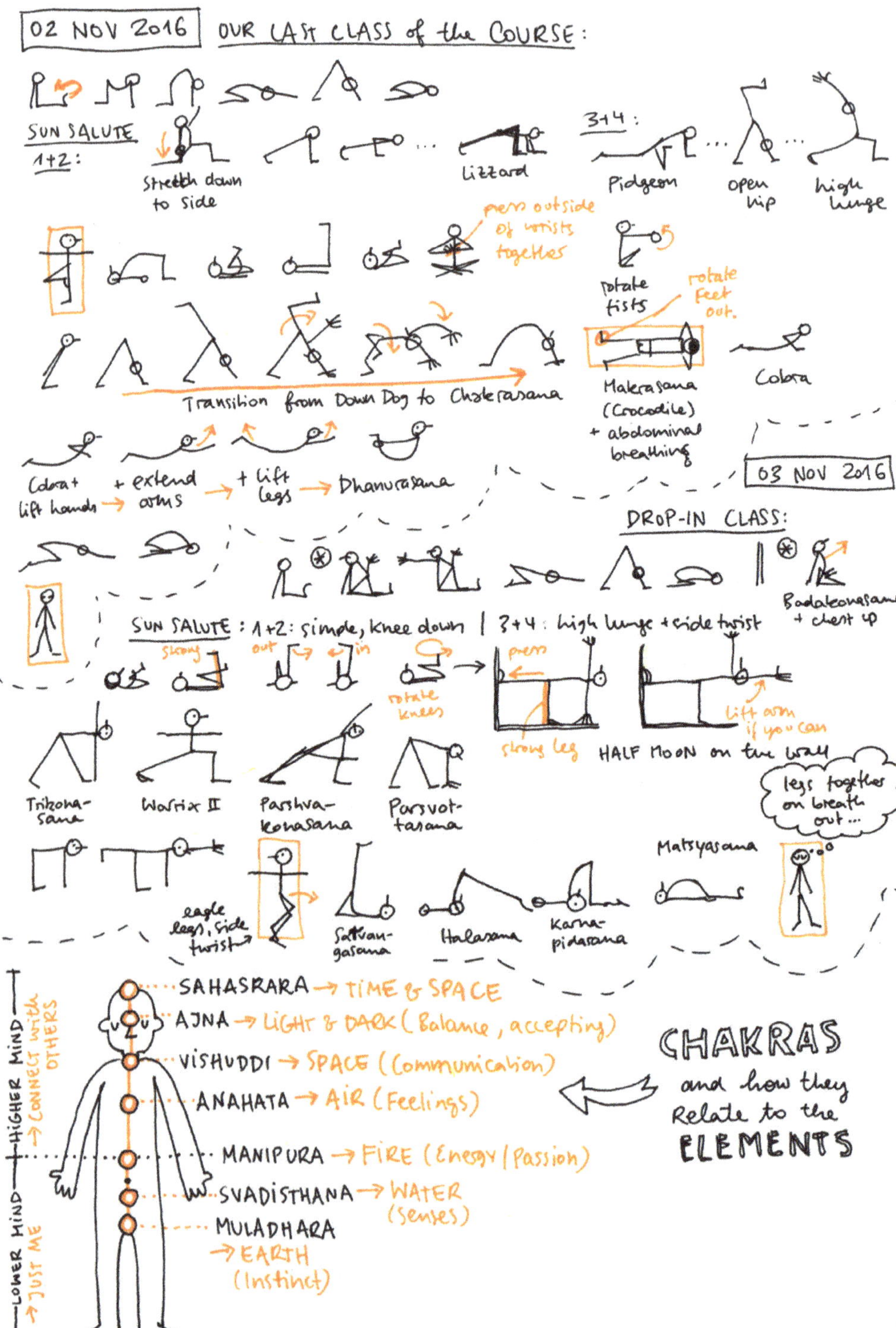

02 NOV 2016
OUR LAST CLASS of the COURSE:

SUN SALUTE
1+2:
Stretch down to side
Lizzard
3+4:
Pidgeon
open hip
high lunge

press outside of wrists together
rotate fists
rotate feet out.
Transition from Down Dog to Chaterasana
Makrasana (Crocodile) + abdominal breathing
Cobra

Cobra + lift hands → + extend arms → + lift legs → Dhanurasana

03 NOV 2016
DROP-IN CLASS:

Badakonasana + chest up
SUN SALUTE : 1+2: simple, knee down | 3+4: high lunge + side twist
strong
out
in
rotate knees
press
strong leg
HALF MOON on the wall
lift arm if you can
legs together on breath out ...

Trikona-sana
Warrix II
Parshva-konasana
Parsvot-tasana

Matsyasana
eagle legs, side twist
Sarvan-gasana
Halasana
Karna-pidasana

HIGHER MIND
→ Connect with OTHERS
LOWER MIND
→ JUST ME

SAHASRARA → TIME & SPACE
AJNA → LIGHT & DARK (Balance, accepting)
VISHUDDI → SPACE (communication)
ANAHATA → AIR (Feelings)
MANIPURA → FIRE (Energy / Passion)
SVADISTHANA → WATER (senses)
MULADHARA → EARTH (Instinct)

CHAKRAS and how they Relate to the ELEMENTS

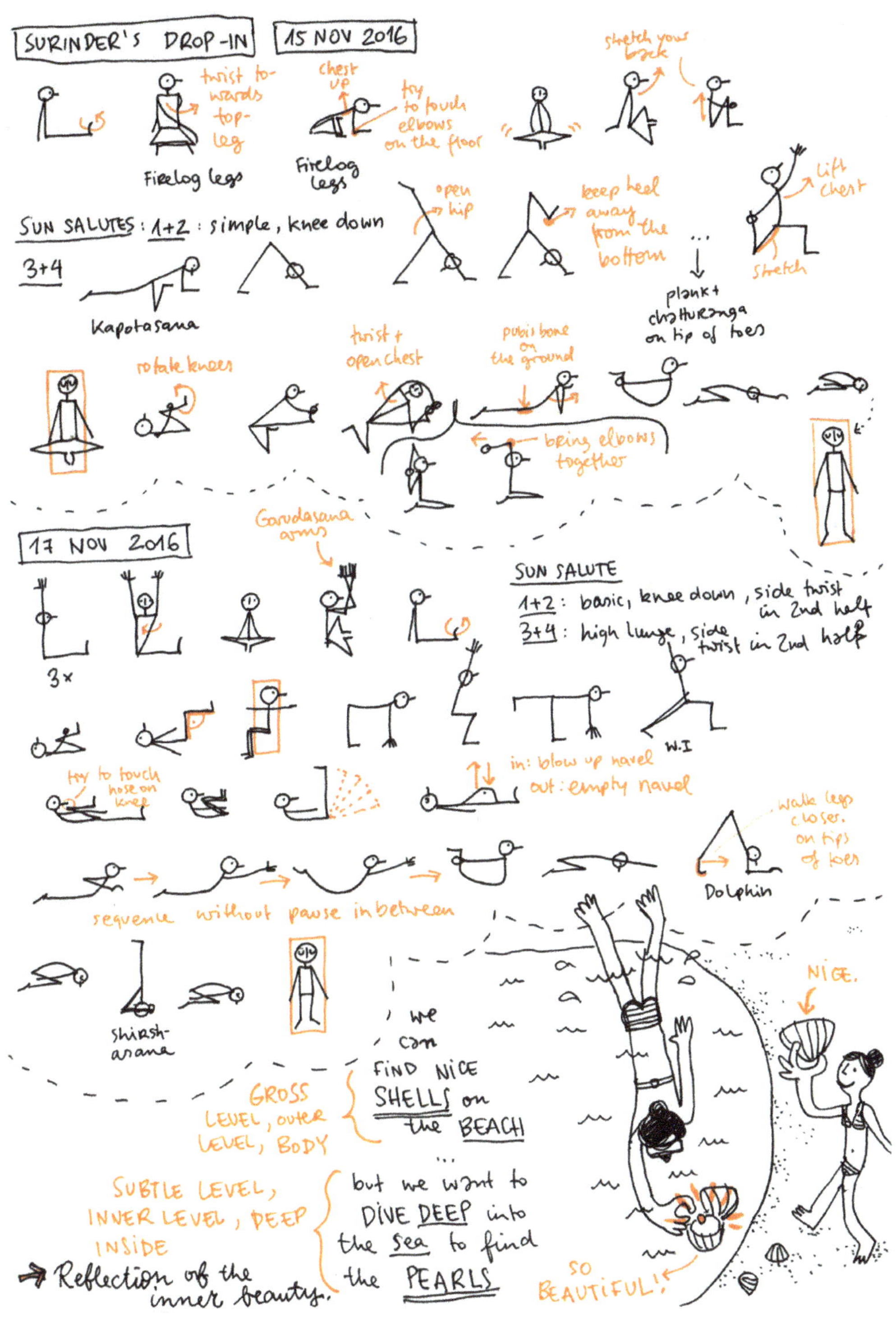

SURINDER'S DROP-IN | 15 NOV 2016
twist towards top-leg
Firelog legs
chest up
try to touch elbows on the floor
Firelog legs
stretch your back
lift chest
stretch
SUN SALUTES : 1+2 : simple, knee down
3+4
Kapotasana
open hip
keep heel away from the bottom
plank + chathuranga on tip of toes
rotate knees
twist + open chest
pubis bone on the ground
bring elbows together
17 NOV 2016
Garudasana arms
SUN SALUTE
1+2: basic, knee down, side twist in 2nd half
3+4: high lunge, side twist in 2nd half
3 x
W.I
try to touch nose on knee
in: blow up navel
out: empty navel
walk legs closer, on tips of toes
Dolphin
sequence without pause inbetween
shirsh-asana
we can FIND NICE SHELLS on the BEACH
NICE.
GROSS LEVEL, OUTER LEVEL, BODY
SUBTLE LEVEL, INNER LEVEL, DEEP INSIDE
but we want to DIVE DEEP into the sea to find the PEARLS
→ Reflection of the inner beauty.
SO BEAUTIFUL!

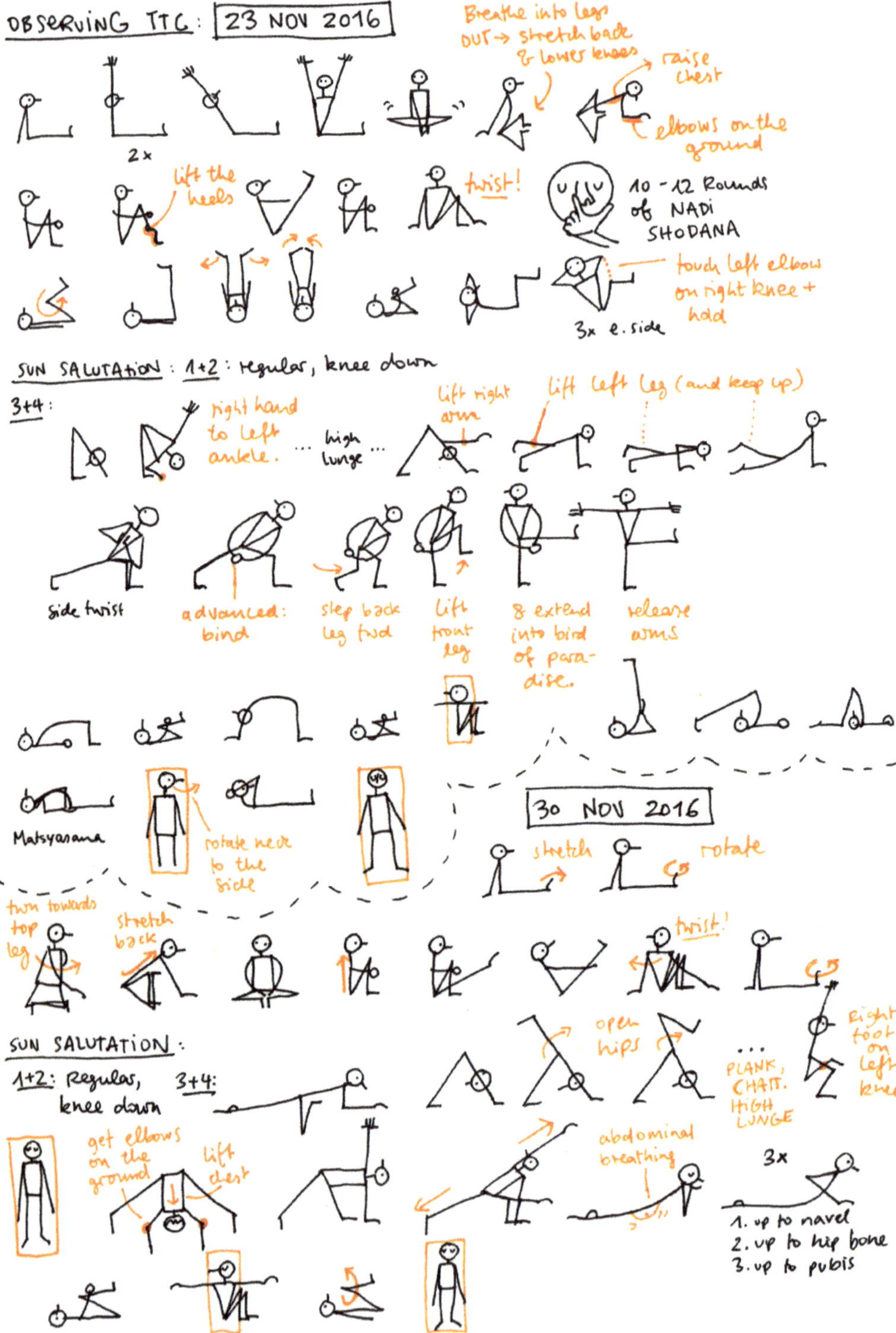

OBSERVING TTC: 23 NOV 2016
2x
Breathe into legs
OUT → stretch back
& lower knees
raise chest
elbows on the ground
lift the heels
twist!
10 - 12 Rounds of NADI SHODANA
touch left elbow on right knee + hold
3x e. side
SUN SALUTATION: 1+2: regular, knee down
3+4:
right hand to left ankle.
... high lunge ...
lift right arm
lift left leg (and keep up)
side twist
advanced: bind
step back leg fwd
lift front leg
& extend into bird of paradise.
release arms
Matsyasana
rotate neck to the side
30 NOV 2016
stretch
rotate
turn towards top leg
stretch back
twist!
SUN SALUTATION:
1+2: Regular, knee down
3+4:
open hips
PLANK, CHATT. HIGH LUNGE
Right foot on left knee
get elbows on the ground
lift chest
abdominal breathing
3x
1. up to navel
2. up to hip bone
3. up to pubis

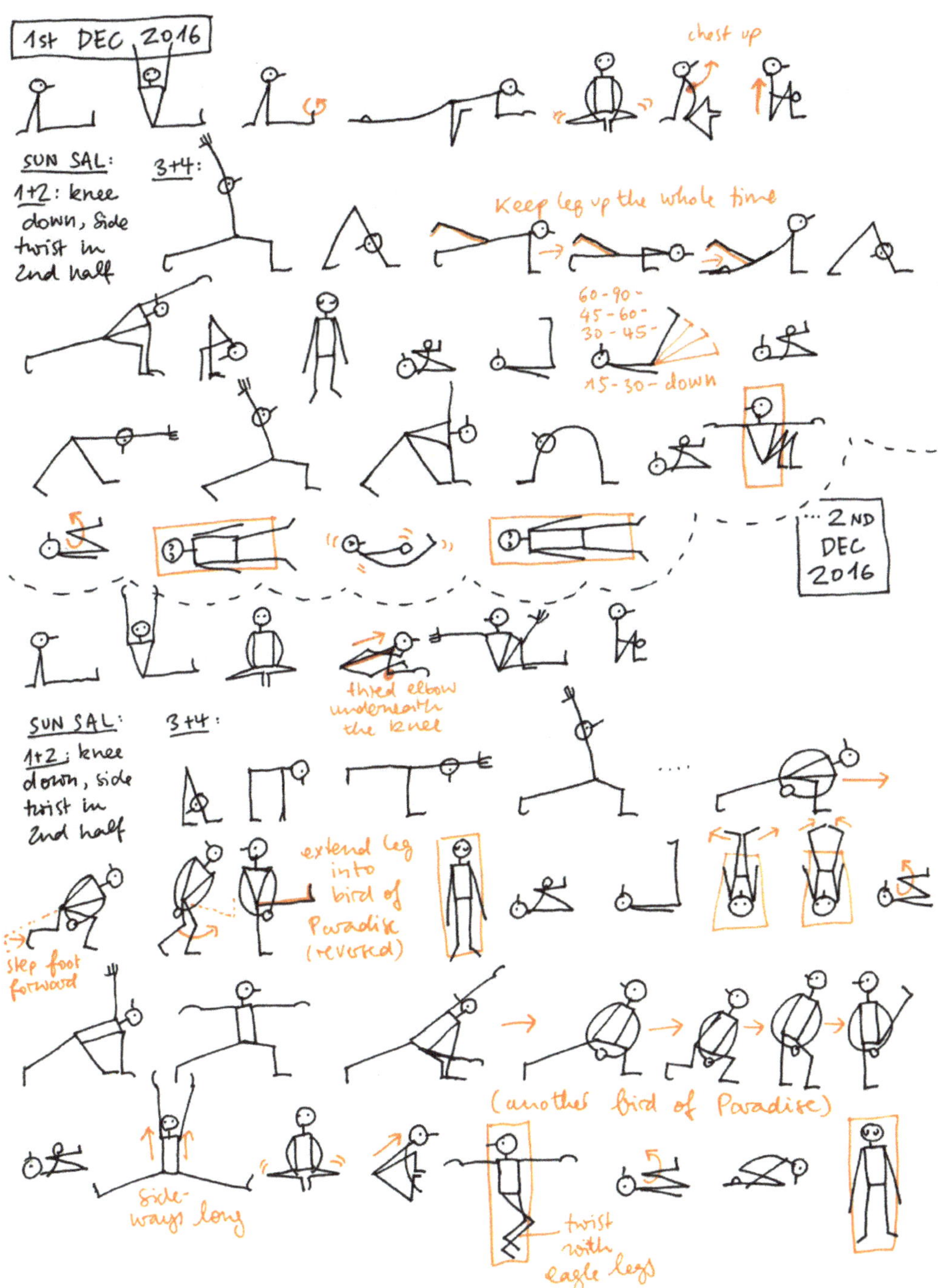

1st DEC 2016

chest up

SUN SAL:
1+2: knee down, Side twist in 2nd half

3+4:

Keep leg up the whole time

60-90-
45-60-
30-45-
15-30- down

... 2ND DEC 2016

third elbow underneath the knee

SUN SAL:
1+2: knee down, side twist in 2nd half

3+4:

extend leg into bird of Paradise (reversed)

...

step foot forward

Side-ways long

(another bird of Paradise)

twist with eagle legs

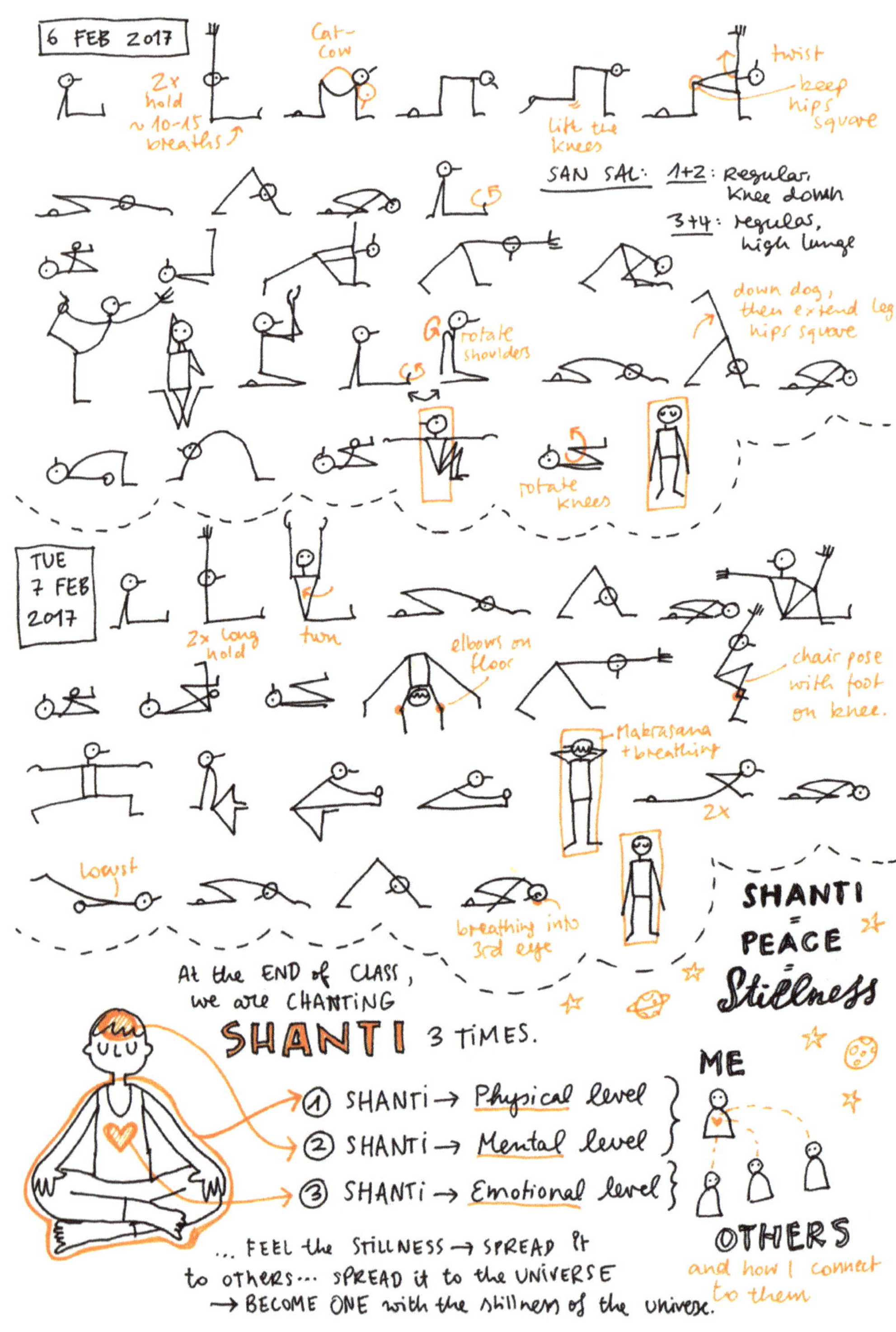
6 FEB 2017
2x hold ~10-15 breaths
Cat-Cow
lift the knees
twist
keep hips square
SAN SAL: 1+2: Regular, knee down
3+4: regular, high lunge
rotate shoulders
down dog, then extend leg, hips square
rotate knees
TUE 7 FEB 2017
2x long hold
turn
elbows on floor
Makrasana + breathing
chair pose with foot on knee
Locust
2x
breathing into 3rd eye
SHANTI = PEACE = Stillness
At the END of CLASS, we are CHANTING SHANTI 3 TIMES.
1 SHANTI → Physical level
2 SHANTI → Mental level
3 SHANTI → Emotional level
ME
OTHERS
and how I connect to them
... FEEL the STILLNESS → SPREAD it to others... SPREAD it to the UNIVERSE → BECOME ONE with the stillness of the universe.
ULU

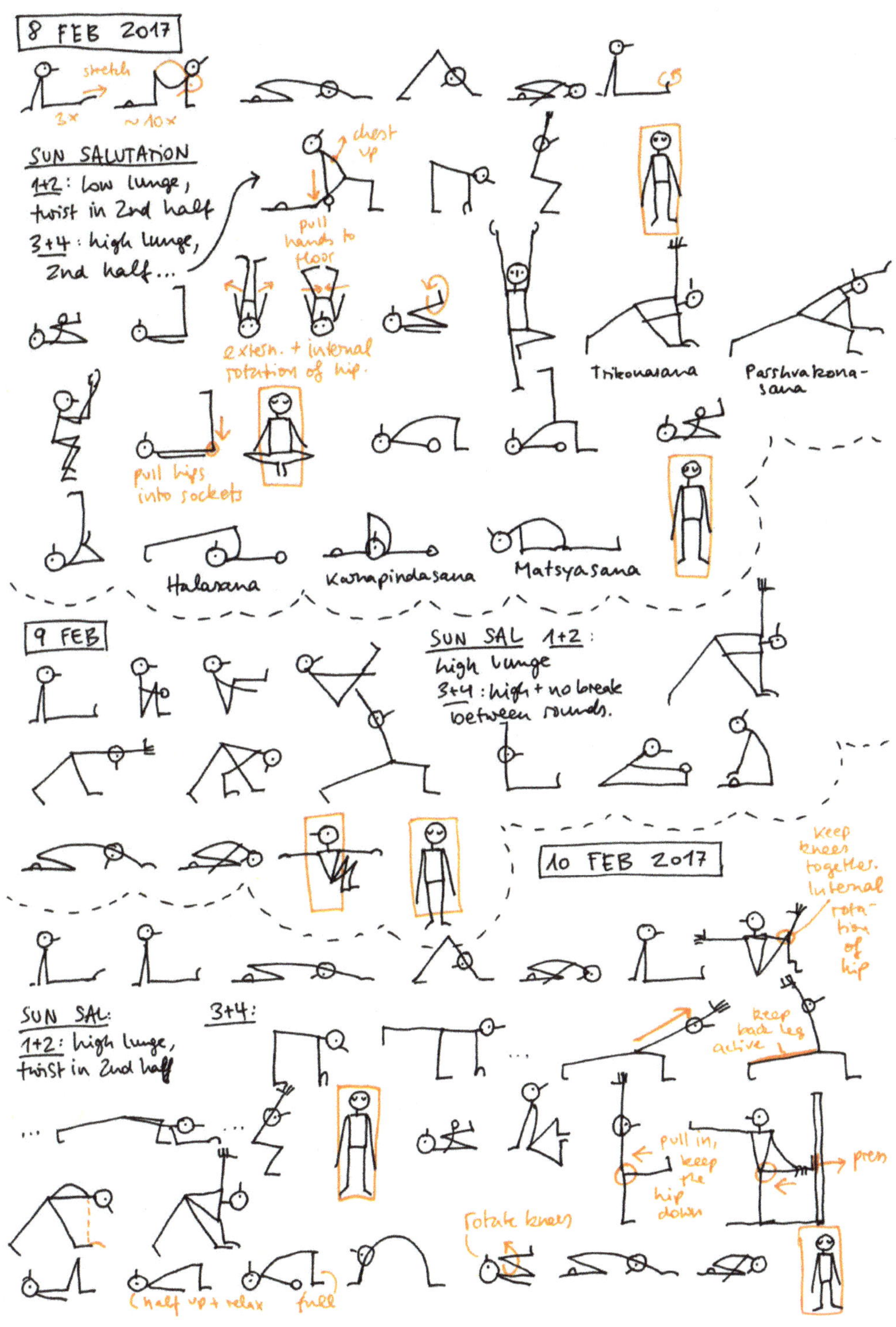
8 FEB 2017
stretch
3x
~10x
SUN SALUTATION
1+2: low lunge,
twist in 2nd half
3+4: high lunge,
2nd half...
chest up
pull hands to floor
extern. + internal rotation of hip.
Trikonasana
Passhvakona-sana
pull hips into sockets
Halasana
Karnapindasana
Matsyasana
9 FEB
SUN SAL 1+2:
high lunge
3+4: high + no break between rounds.
10 FEB 2017
keep knees together. Internal rotation of hip
keep back leg active
SUN SAL:
1+2: high lunge, twist in 2nd half
3+4:
pull in, keep the hip down
push
rotate knees
half up + relax
free

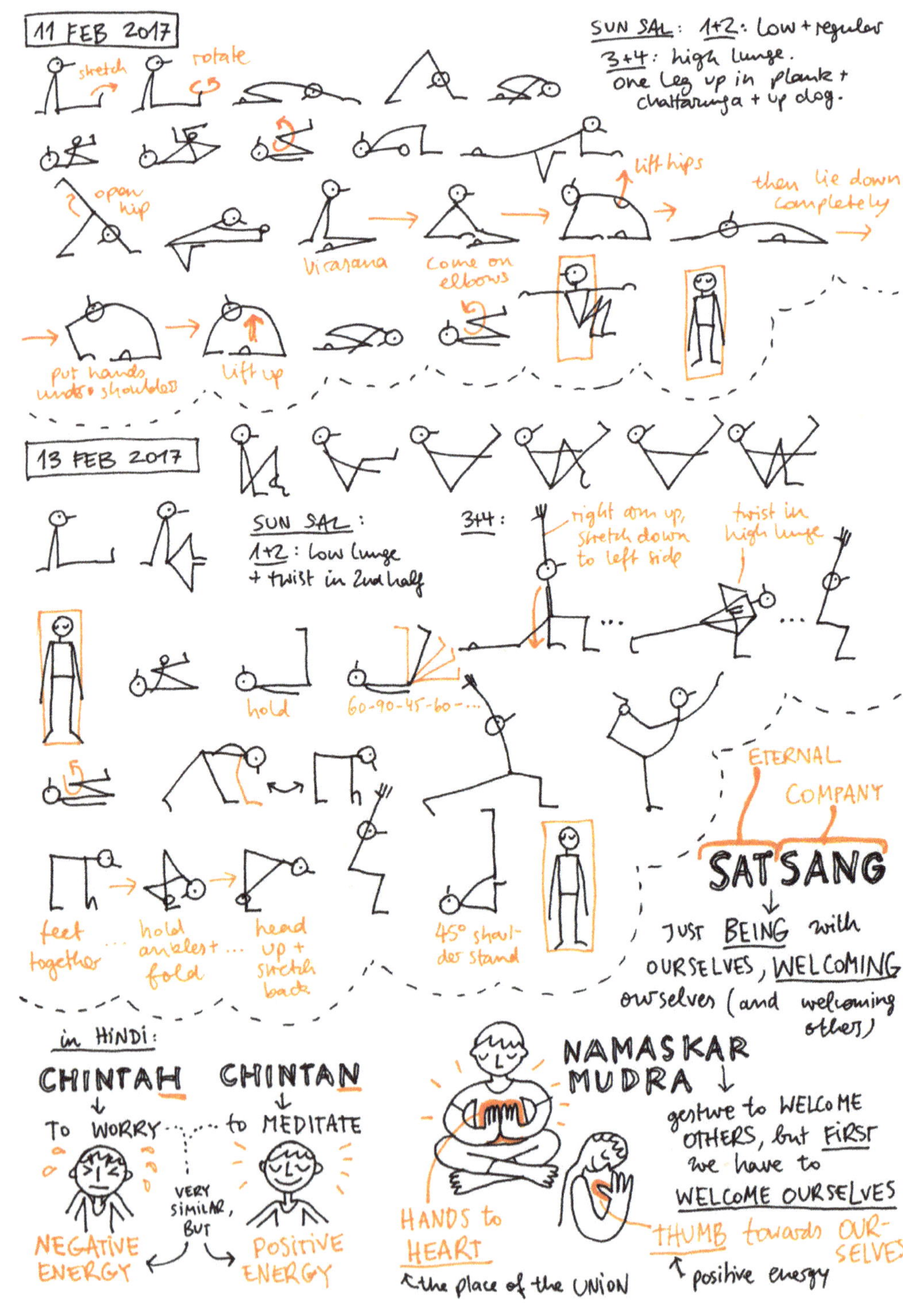

11 FEB 2017
stretch
rotate
SUN SAL: 1+2: low + regular
3+4: high lunge.
one leg up in plank +
chatturanga + up dog.
open hip
Virasana
come on elbows
lift hips
then lie down completely
put hands under shoulders
lift up
13 FEB 2017
SUN SAL:
1+2: low lunge
+ twist in 2nd half
3+4:
right arm up, stretch down to left side
twist in high lunge
hold
60-90-45-60-...
feet together
hold ankles + ... fold
head up + stretch back
45° shoulder stand
ETERNAL COMPANY
SATSANG
JUST BEING with OURSELVES, WELCOMING ourselves (and welcoming others)
in HINDI:
CHINTAH
to WORRY
NEGATIVE ENERGY
CHINTAN
to MEDITATE
VERY SIMILAR, BUT
POSITIVE ENERGY
NAMASKAR MUDRA
gesture to WELCOME OTHERS, but FIRST we have to WELCOME OURSELVES
HANDS to HEART
the place of the UNION
THUMB towards OUR-SELVES
positive energy

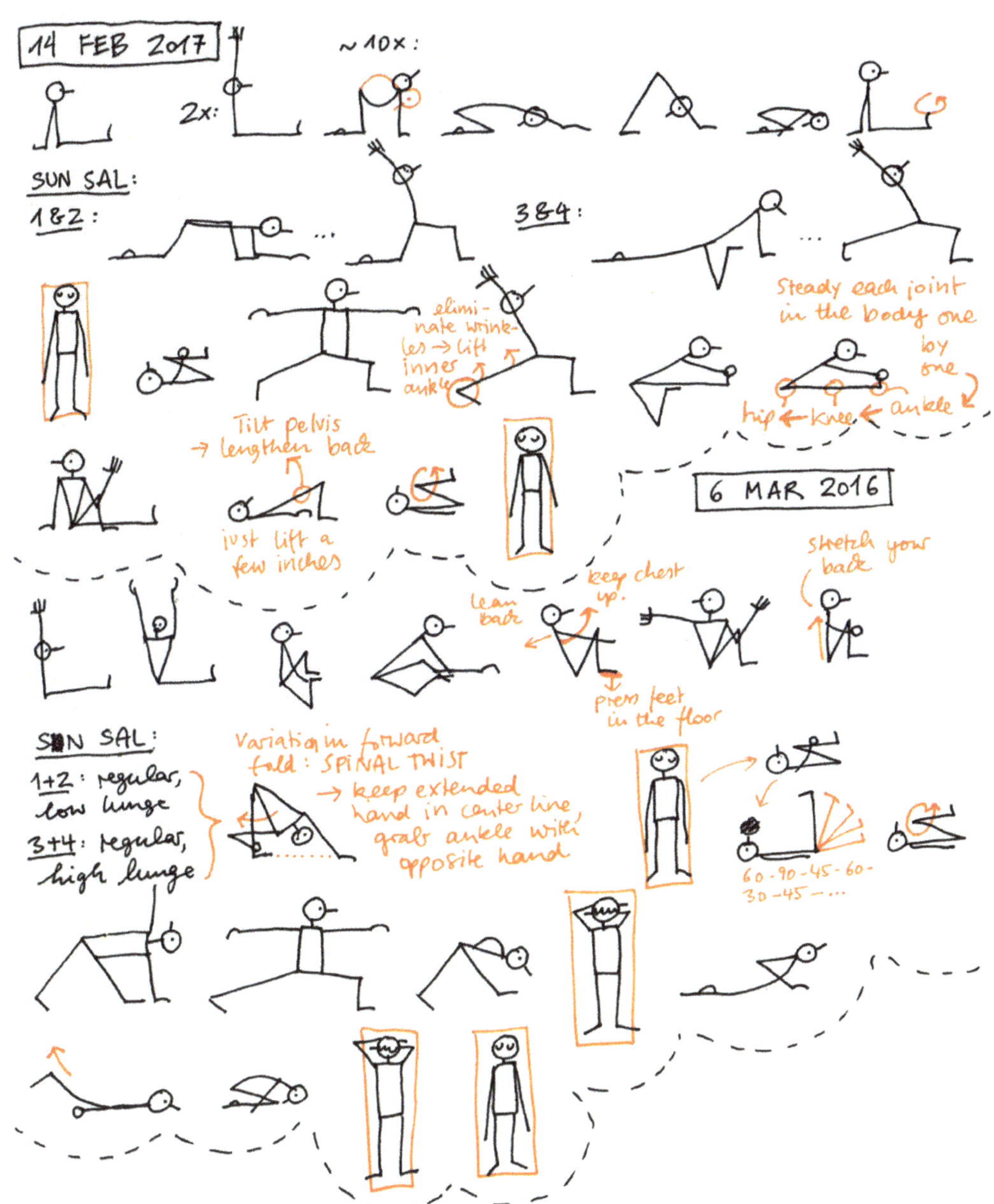

14 FEB 2017
~ 10x:
2x:
SUN SAL:
1 & 2:   ...   3 & 4:   ...
elimi-
nate wrink-
les → lift
inner
ankle
Steady each joint
in the body one
by
one
hip ← knee ← ankle
Tilt pelvis
→ lengthen back
just lift a
few inches
6 MAR 2016
keep chest
up.
lean
back
stretch your
back
press feet
in the floor
SUN SAL:
1+2: regular,
low lunge
3+4: regular,
high lunge
Variation in forward
fold: SPINAL TWIST
→ keep extended
hand in center line,
grab ankle with
opposite hand
60-90-45-60-
30-45-...

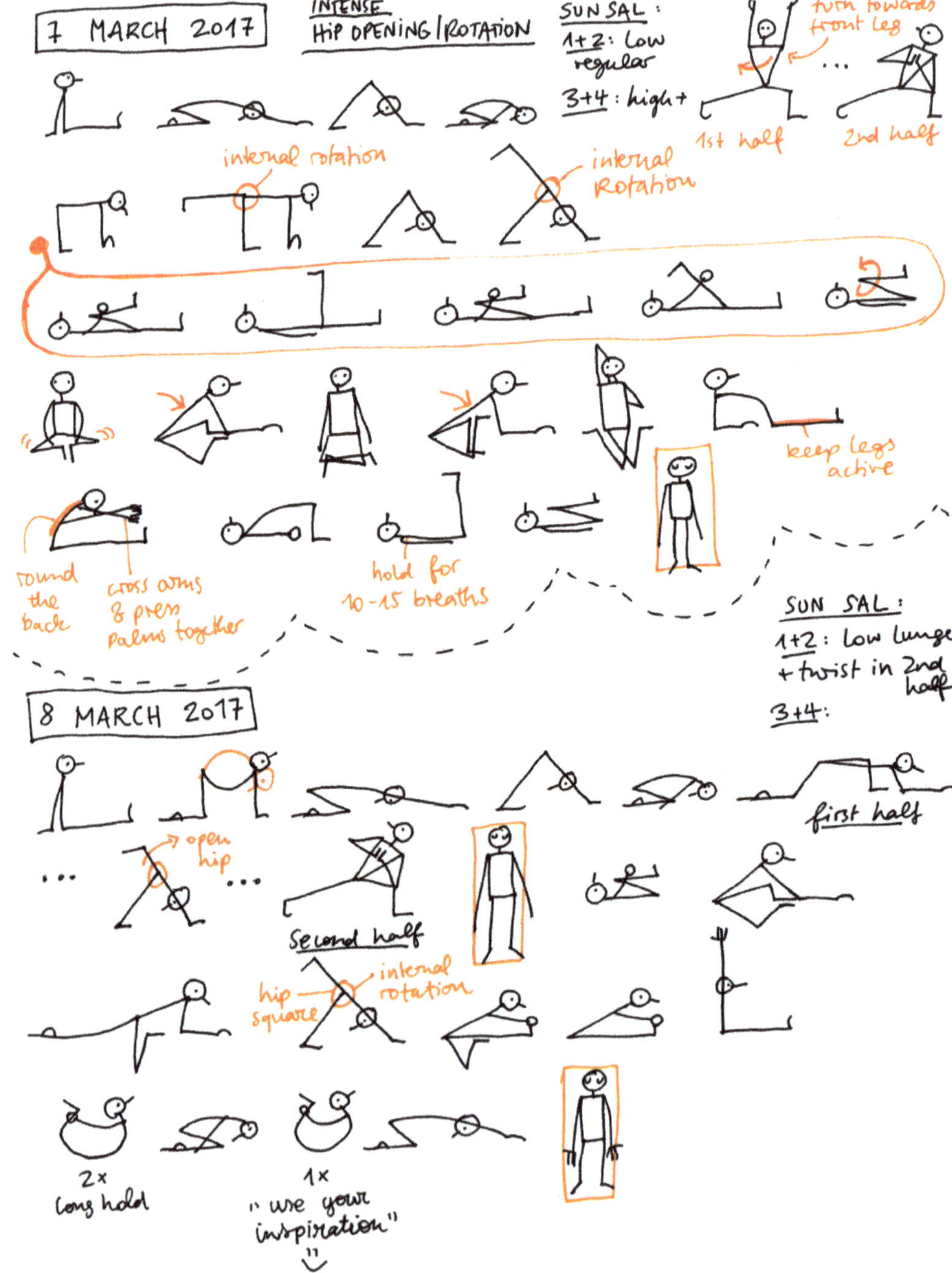

7 MARCH 2017
INTENSE
HIP OPENING / ROTATION
SUN SAL:
1+2: Low regular
3+4: high+
turn towards front leg
...
1st half
2nd half
internal rotation
internal rotation
keep legs active
round the back
cross arms & press palms together
hold for 10-15 breaths
SUN SAL:
1+2: Low lunge + twist in 2nd half
3+4:
8 MARCH 2017
open hip
...
...
first half
Second half
hip square
internal rotation
2x long hold
1x "use your inspiration"

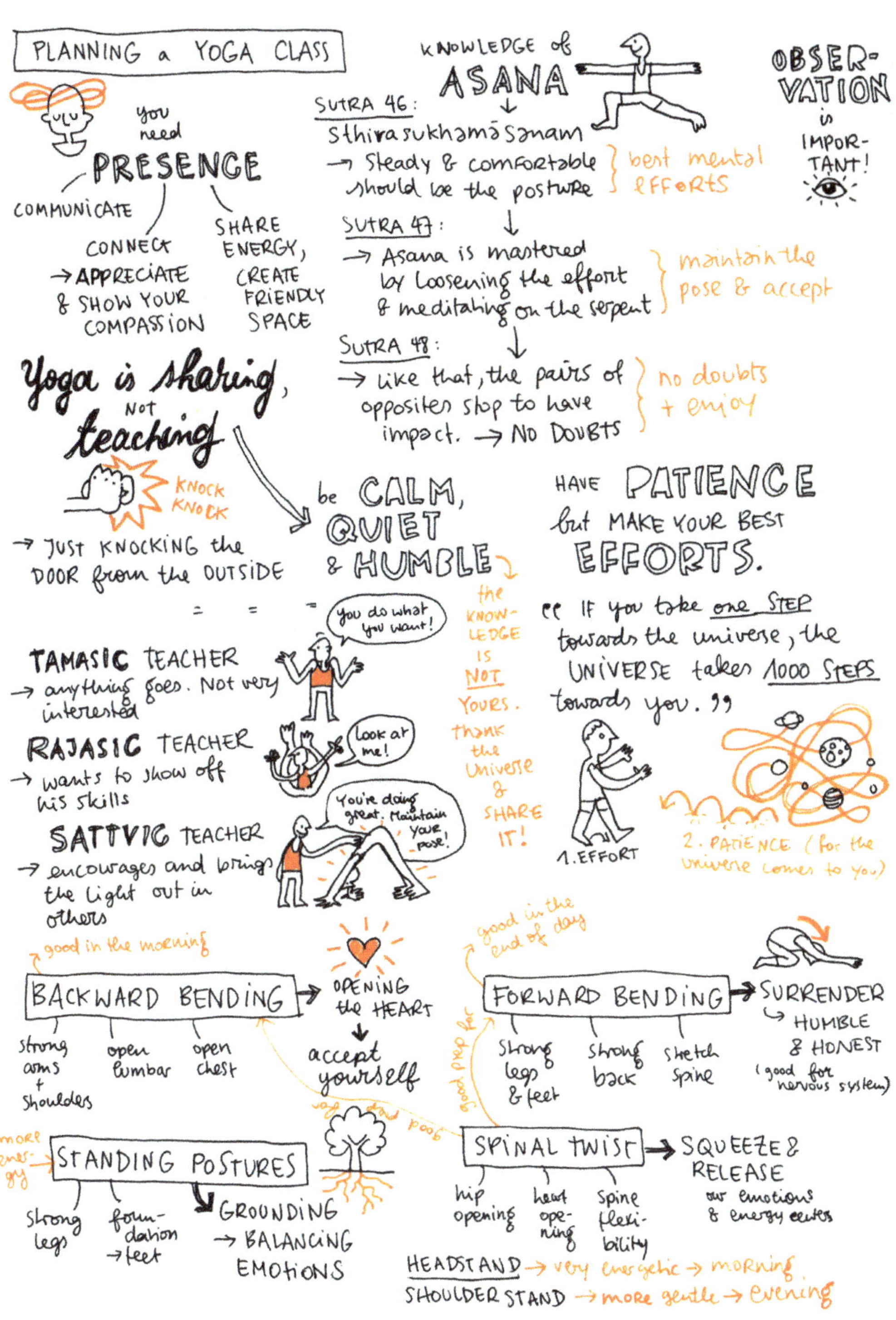

PLANNING a YOGA CLASS

you need
PRESENCE

COMMUNICATE
CONNECT
→ APPRECIATE & SHOW YOUR COMPASSION
SHARE ENERGY, CREATE FRIENDLY SPACE

Yoga is sharing, NOT teaching

KNOCK KNOCK
→ JUST KNOCKING the DOOR from the OUTSIDE

TAMASIC TEACHER
→ anything goes. Not very interested

RAJASIC TEACHER
→ wants to show off his skills

SATTVIC TEACHER
→ encourages and brings the light out in others

good in the morning

BACKWARD BENDING → OPENING the HEART
accept yourself

strong arms + shoulders
open lumbar
open chest

more energy → STANDING POSTURES
strong legs
foun-dation → feet
→ GROUNDING → BALANCING EMOTIONS

KNOWLEDGE of ASANA

SUTRA 46:
Sthira sukham āsanam
→ Steady & comfortable should be the posture
} best mental efforts

SUTRA 47:
→ Asana is mastered by loosening the effort & meditating on the serpent
} maintain the pose & accept

SUTRA 48:
→ like that, the pairs of opposites stop to have impact. → NO DOUBTS
} no doubts + enjoy

be CALM, QUIET & HUMBLE

you do what you want!
look at me!
You're doing great. Maintain your pose!

the KNOWLEDGE IS NOT YOURS. thank the universe & SHARE IT!

OBSER-VATION is IMPORTANT!

HAVE PATIENCE but MAKE YOUR BEST EFFORTS.

"If you take one STEP towards the universe, the UNIVERSE takes 1000 STEPS towards you."

1. EFFORT
2. PATIENCE (for the universe comes to you)

good in the end of day
good prep for

FORWARD BENDING → SURRENDER
↳ HUMBLE & HONEST (good for nervous system)

strong legs & feet
strong back
stretch spine

SPINAL TWIST → SQUEEZE & RELEASE
our emotions & energy centers

hip opening
heart opening
spine flexi-bility

HEADSTAND → very energetic → morning
SHOULDER STAND → more gentle → evening

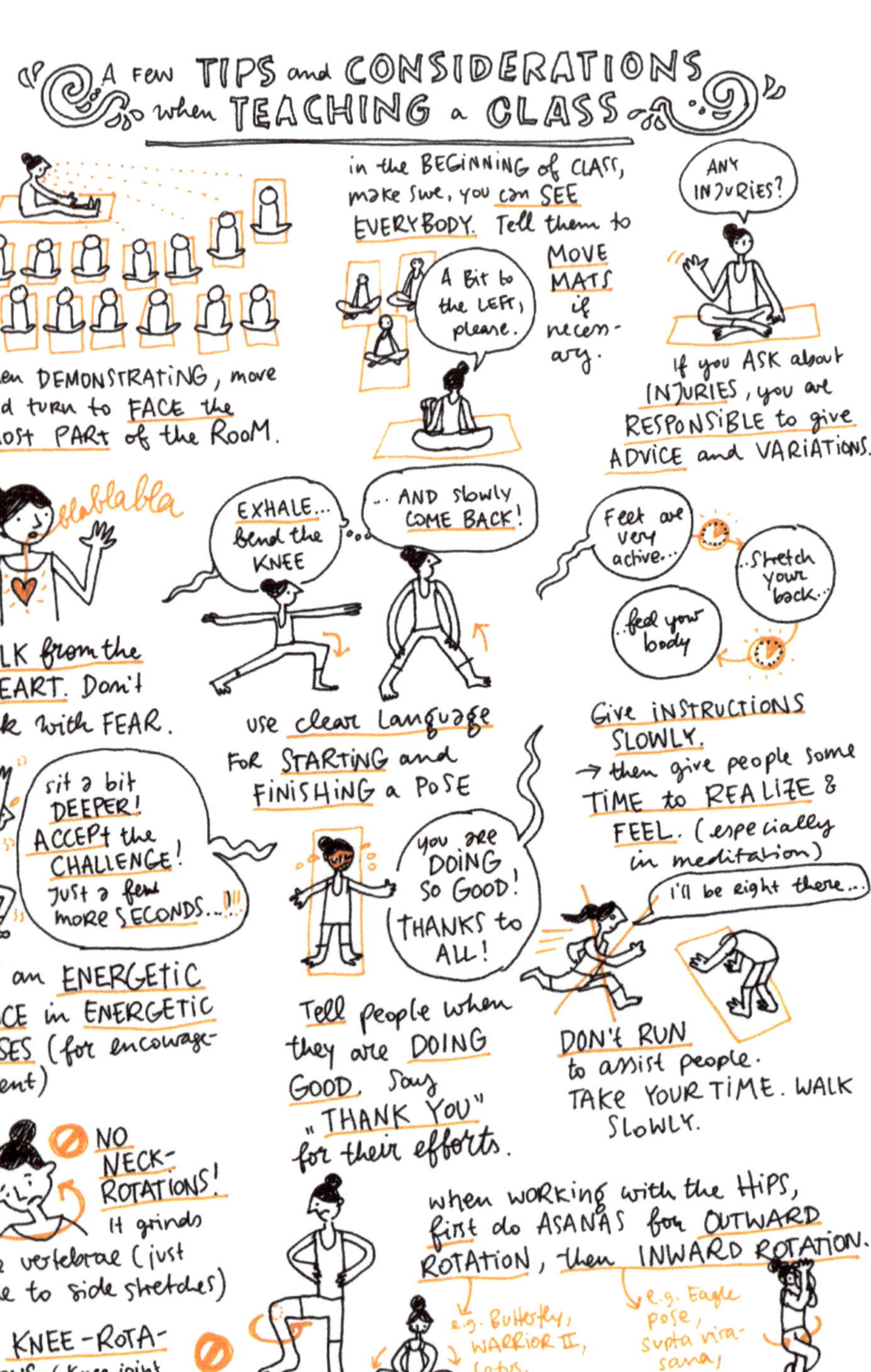

A few TIPS and CONSIDERATIONS when TEACHING a CLASS

when DEMONSTRATING, move and turn to FACE the Most PART of the RooM.

in the BEGINNING of CLASS, make sure, you can SEE EVERYBODY. Tell them to MOVE MATS if necessary.
A Bit to the LEFT, please.

ANY INJURIES?

If you ASK about INJURIES, you are RESPONSIBLE to give ADVICE and VARIATIONS.

blablabla
TALK from the HEART. Don't talk with FEAR.

EXHALE... Bend the KNEE
... AND slowly COME BACK!
use clear language for STARTING and FINISHING a POSE

Feet are very active...
..Stretch your back...
..feel your body
Give INSTRUCTIONS SLOWLY.
→ then give people some TIME to REALIZE & FEEL. (especially in meditation)

sit a bit DEEPER! ACCEPT the CHALLENGE! Just a few more SECONDS...!!
USE an ENERGETIC VOICE in ENERGETIC POSES (for encouragement)

you are DOING SO GOOD! THANKS to ALL!
Tell people when they are DOING GOOD. Say „THANK YOU" for their efforts.

I'll be right there...
DON'T RUN to assist people. TAKE YOUR TIME. WALK SLOWLY.

NO NECK-ROTATIONS! It grinds the vertebrae (just side to side stretches)
NO KNEE-ROTA-TIONS (Knee joint is just for bending)

when WORKING with the HIPS, first do ASANAS for OUTWARD ROTATION, then INWARD ROTATION.
e.g. Butterfly, WARRIOR II, Lotus, PARSHVOKONA-SANA,...
e.g. Eagle pose, supta vira-sana, etc...

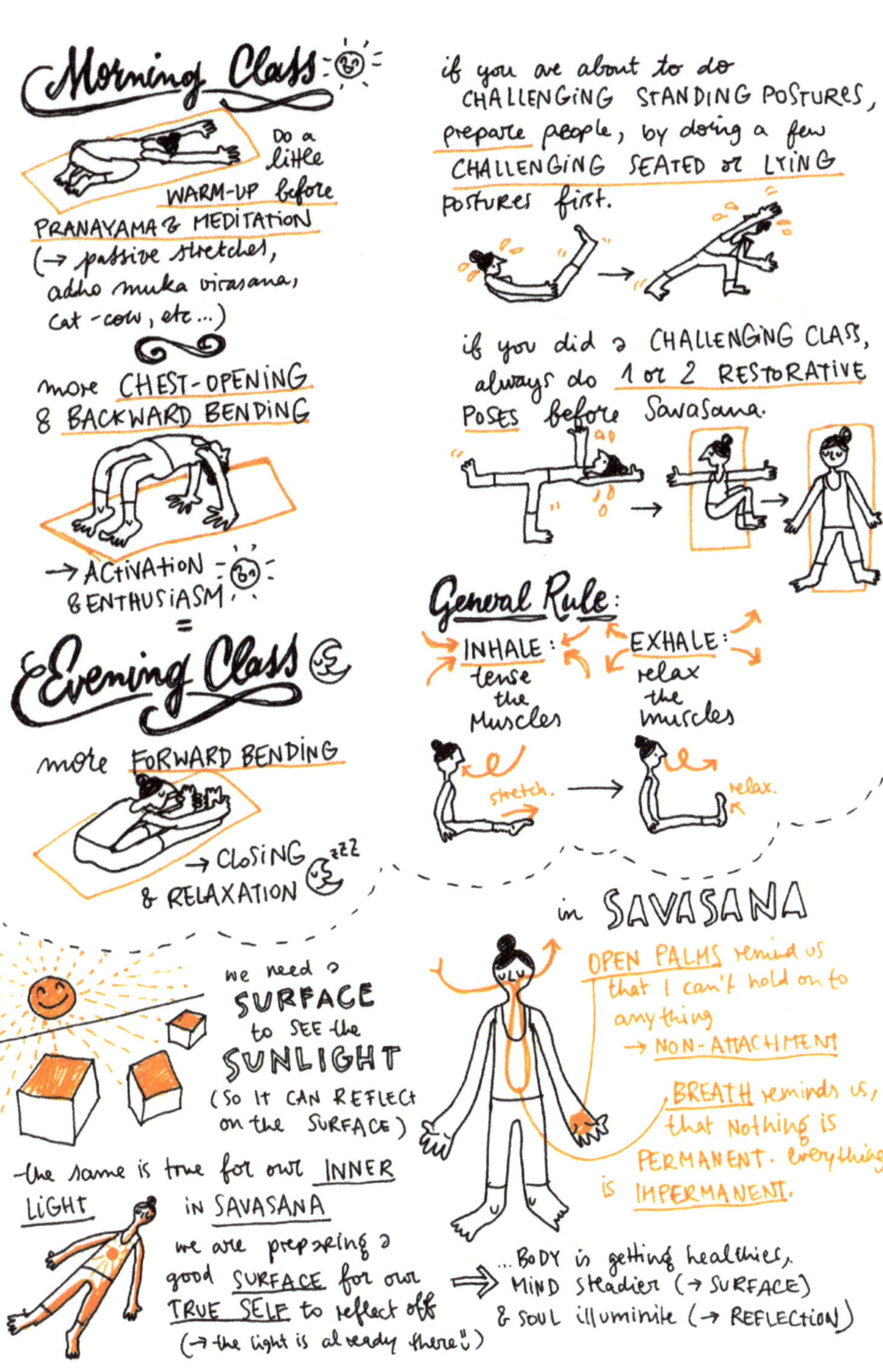

Morning Class

Do a little WARM-UP before PRANAYAMA & MEDITATION
(→ passive stretches, adho muka virasana, cat-cow, etc...)

more CHEST-OPENING & BACKWARD BENDING

→ ACTIVATION & ENTHUSIASM
=

Evening Class

more FORWARD BENDING

→ CLOSING & RELAXATION

if you are about to do CHALLENGING STANDING POSTURES, prepare people, by doing a few CHALLENGING SEATED or LYING postures first.

if you did a CHALLENGING CLASS, always do 1 or 2 RESTORATIVE POSES before Savasana.

General Rule:

→ INHALE: tense the Muscles

EXHALE: relax the muscles

stretch. → relax.

we need a SURFACE to SEE the SUNLIGHT
(so it can REFLECT on the SURFACE)

the same is true for our INNER LIGHT in SAVASANA
we are preparing a good SURFACE for our TRUE SELF to reflect off
(→ the light is already there!!)

in SAVASANA

OPEN PALMS remind us that I can't hold on to anything
→ NON-ATTACHMENT

BREATH reminds us, that nothing is PERMANENT. everything is IMPERMANENT.

...BODY is getting healthier, MIND steadier (→ SURFACE) & soul illuminate (→ REFLECTION)

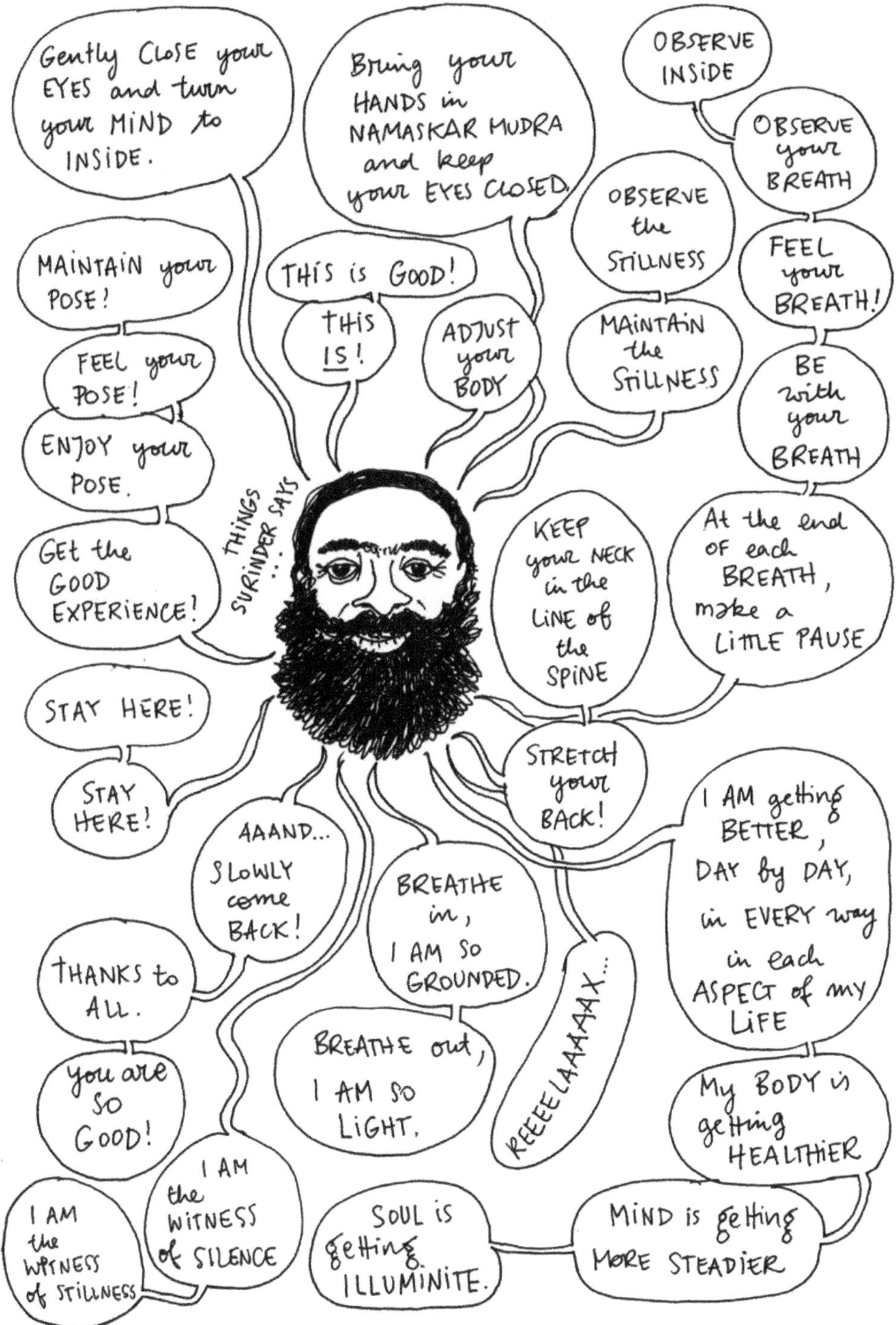

Gently CLOSE your EYES and turn your MIND to INSIDE.
Bring your HANDS in NAMASKAR MUDRA and keep your EYES CLOSED.
OBSERVE INSIDE
OBSERVE your BREATH
OBSERVE the STILLNESS
FEEL your BREATH!
MAINTAIN your POSE!
THIS is GOOD!
THIS IS!
ADJUST your BODY
MAINTAIN the STILLNESS
BE with your BREATH
FEEL your POSE!
ENJOY your POSE.
THINGS SURINDER SAYS...
KEEP your NECK in the LINE of the SPINE
At the end of each BREATH, make a LITTLE PAUSE
GET the GOOD EXPERIENCE!
STRETCH your BACK!
STAY HERE!
STAY HERE!
I AM getting BETTER, DAY by DAY, in EVERY way in each ASPECT of my LIFE
AAAND... SLOWLY come BACK!
BREATHE in, I AM SO GROUNDED.
THANKS to ALL.
REEEEE LAAAAAX...
BREATHE out, I AM SO LIGHT.
My BODY is getting HEALTHIER
you are SO GOOD!
I AM the WITNESS of STILLNESS
I AM the WITNESS of SILENCE
SOUL is getting ILLUMINITE.
MIND is getting MORE STEADIER

YOGA DROP-IN CLASSES

TAUGHT BY
ASHISH SHARMA

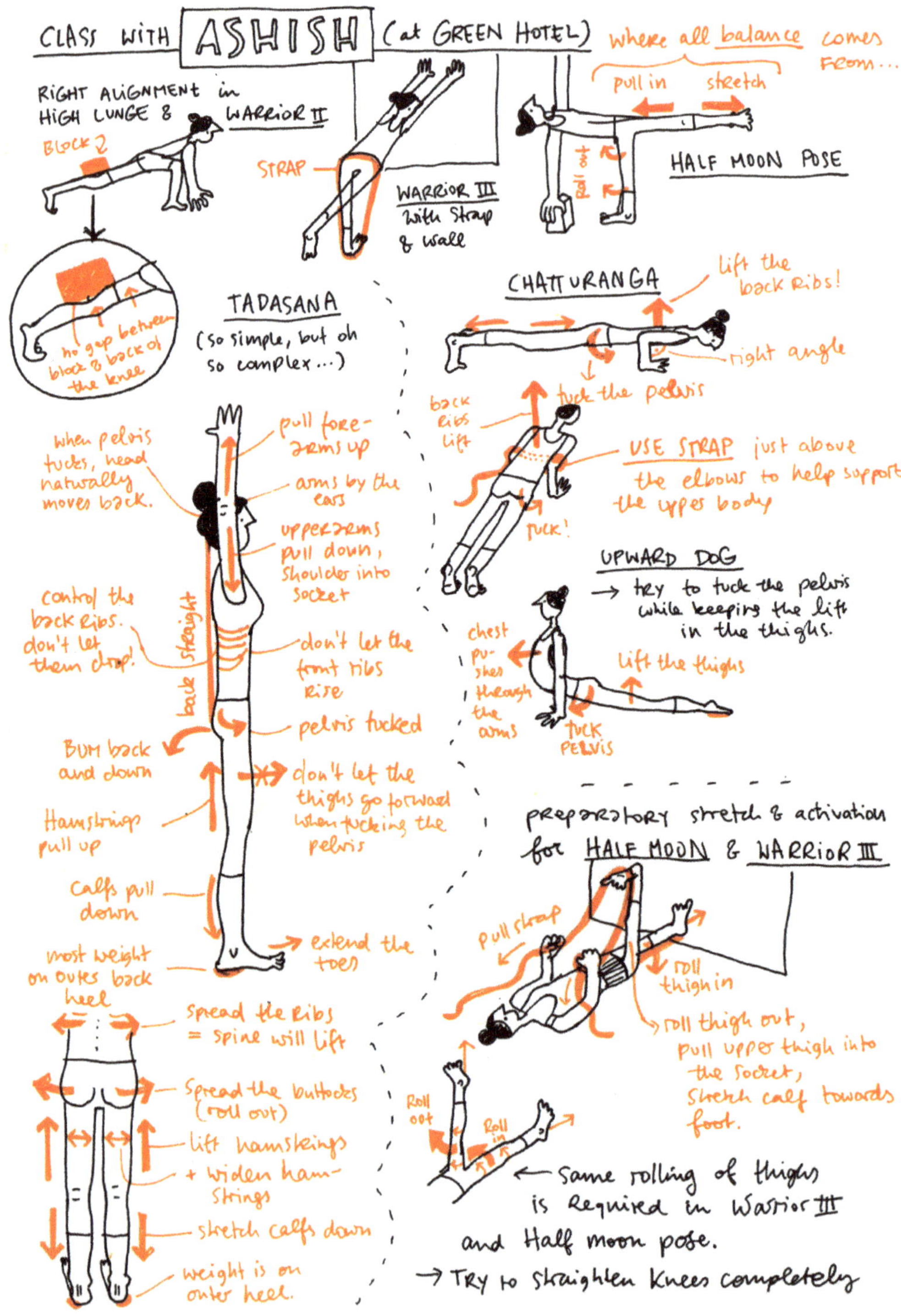

CLASS WITH ASHISH (at GREEN HOTEL)
RIGHT ALIGNMENT in HIGH LUNGE & WARRIOR II
BLOCK 2
STRAP
WARRIOR III with strap & wall
where all balance comes from...
pull in   stretch
Roll out
HALF MOON POSE
no gap between block & back of the knee
TADASANA
(so simple, but oh so complex...)
CHATTURANGA
lift the back ribs!
right angle
back ribs lift
tuck the pelvis
USE STRAP just above the elbows to help support the upper body
tuck!
UPWARD DOG
→ try to tuck the pelvis while keeping the lift in the thighs.
lift the thighs
chest pushes through the arms
tuck pelvis
when pelvis tucks, head naturally moves back.
pull fore-arms up
arms by the ears
upper arms pull down, shoulder into socket
back straight
control the back ribs. don't let them drop!
don't let the front ribs rise
pelvis tucked
BUM back and down
don't let the thighs go forward when tucking the pelvis
Hamstrings pull up
Calfs pull down
most weight on outer back heel
extend the toes
spread the ribs = spine will lift
spread the buttocks (roll out)
lift hamstrings + widen ham-strings
stretch calfs down
weight is on outer heel.
preparatory stretch & activation for HALF MOON & WARRIOR III
pull strap
roll thigh in
roll thigh out, pull upper thigh into the socket, stretch calf towards foot.
Roll out
Roll in
← same rolling of thighs is required in Warrior III and Half moon pose.
→ TRY to straighten knees completely

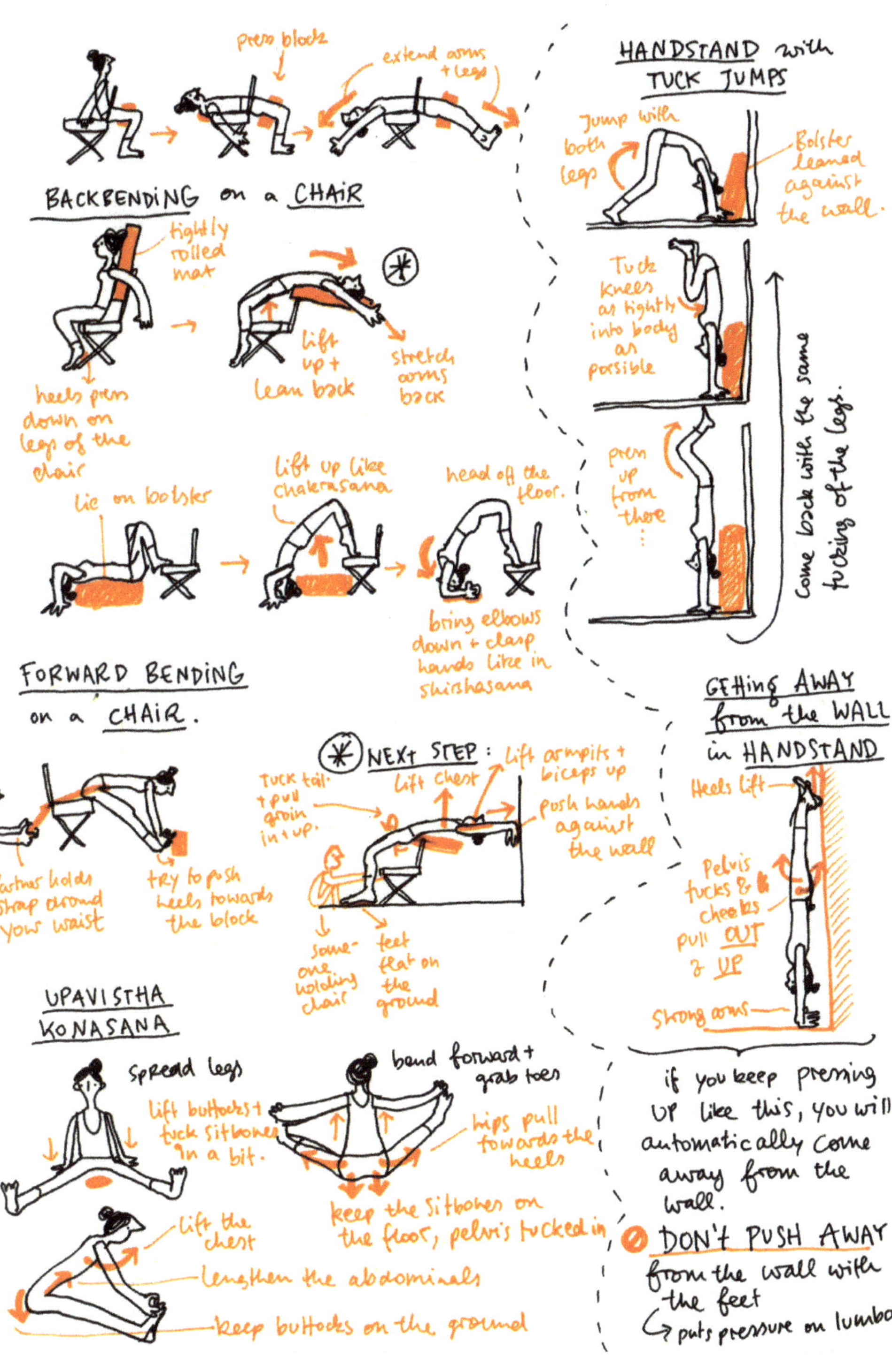

press block
extend arms + legs
HANDSTAND with TUCK JUMPS
Jump with both legs
Bolster leaned against the wall.
BACKBENDING on a CHAIR
tightly rolled mat
*
Tuck knees as tightly into body as possible
heels press down on legs of the chair
lift up + lean back
stretch arms back
lie on bolster
Lift up like chakrasana
head off the floor.
press up from there...
Come back with the same tucking of the legs.
bring elbows down + clasp hands like in shirshasana
FORWARD BENDING on a CHAIR.
*NEXT STEP: Lift armpits + biceps up
Lift chest
GETTING AWAY from the WALL in HANDSTAND
Tuck tail + pull groin in + up.
push hands against the wall
Heels lift
Partner holds strap around your waist
try to push heels towards the block
Pelvis tucks & cheeks pull OUT & UP
some-one holding chair
feet flat on the ground
strong arms
UPAVISTHA KONASANA
spread legs
bend forward + grab toes
if you keep pressing UP like this, you will automatically come away from the wall.
lift buttocks + tuck sitbones in a bit.
hips pull towards the heels
lift the chest
keep the sitbones on the floor, pelvis tucked in
DON'T PUSH AWAY from the wall with the feet
lengthen the abdominals
keep buttocks on the ground
puts pressure on lumbar

WARMING UP ARMS & SHOULDERS

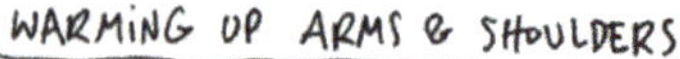

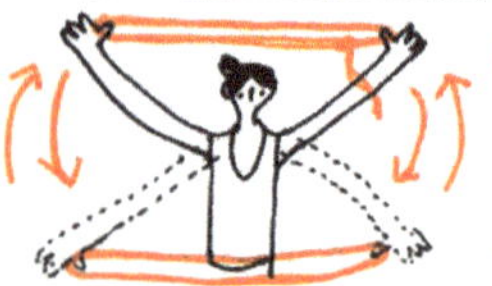

move front & back 15 times.
= keep strap tight. Don't lift shoulders

try to straighten your arms.

press block between the heels of your palms

strap shoulder-width around your wrists.

"Try to break the strap."

HANDS & WRISTS
in

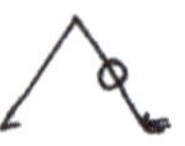 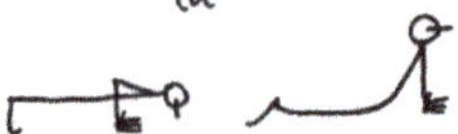

DOWN DOG   CHATTU-RANGA   &   UPWARD DOG

where is the pressure in your hands in each of the postures.

→ Does it change between postures ... and how?

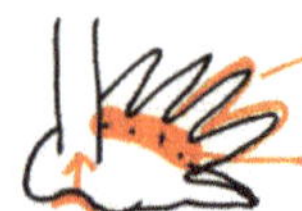

ideally, focus on 2nd + 3rd finger.

pressure should be on the KNUCKLES

Keep the ARCH in the heel of your wrist.

Protect the WRIST!

spread the finger really wide

Press thumb down and move away from the body to rotate it IN A BIT. helps to press it down more.

you want the hand be so active—that all the METACARPALS to SHOW

TURNING your FOOT for WARRIOR II

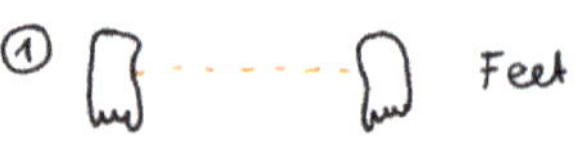

①   Feet parallel

②   first, turn around the heel for 45°

③   then, turn around the mound for the other 45°

like that, the heel will end up in line with the arch.

Avoiding KNEE PAIN in WARRIOR I

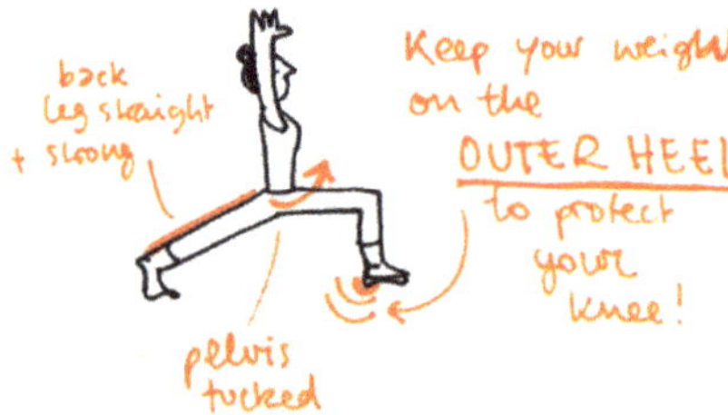

back leg straight + strong

pelvis tucked

Keep your weight on the OUTER HEEL to protect your knee!

ASSISTED SIDE TWIST

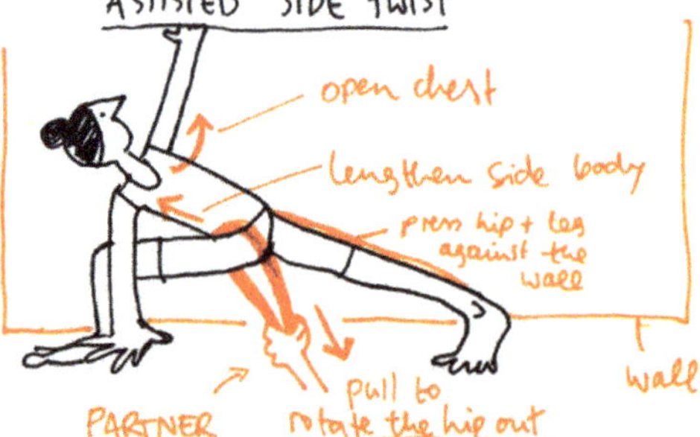

open chest

lengthen side body

press hip + leg against the wall

PARTNER

pull to rotate the hip out

wall

Stretching the LOWER BACK

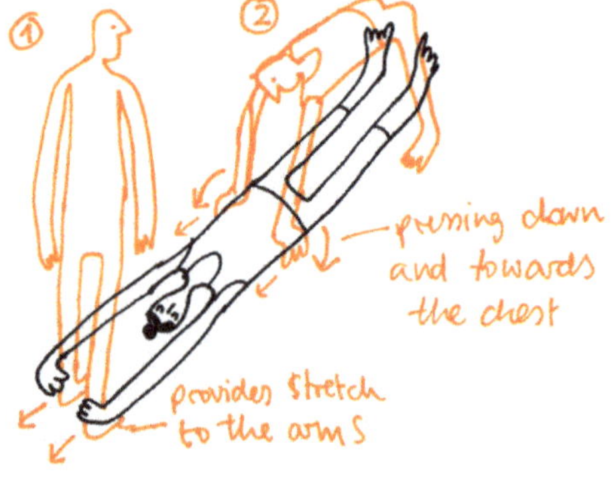

①   ②

pressing down and towards the chest

provides stretch to the arms

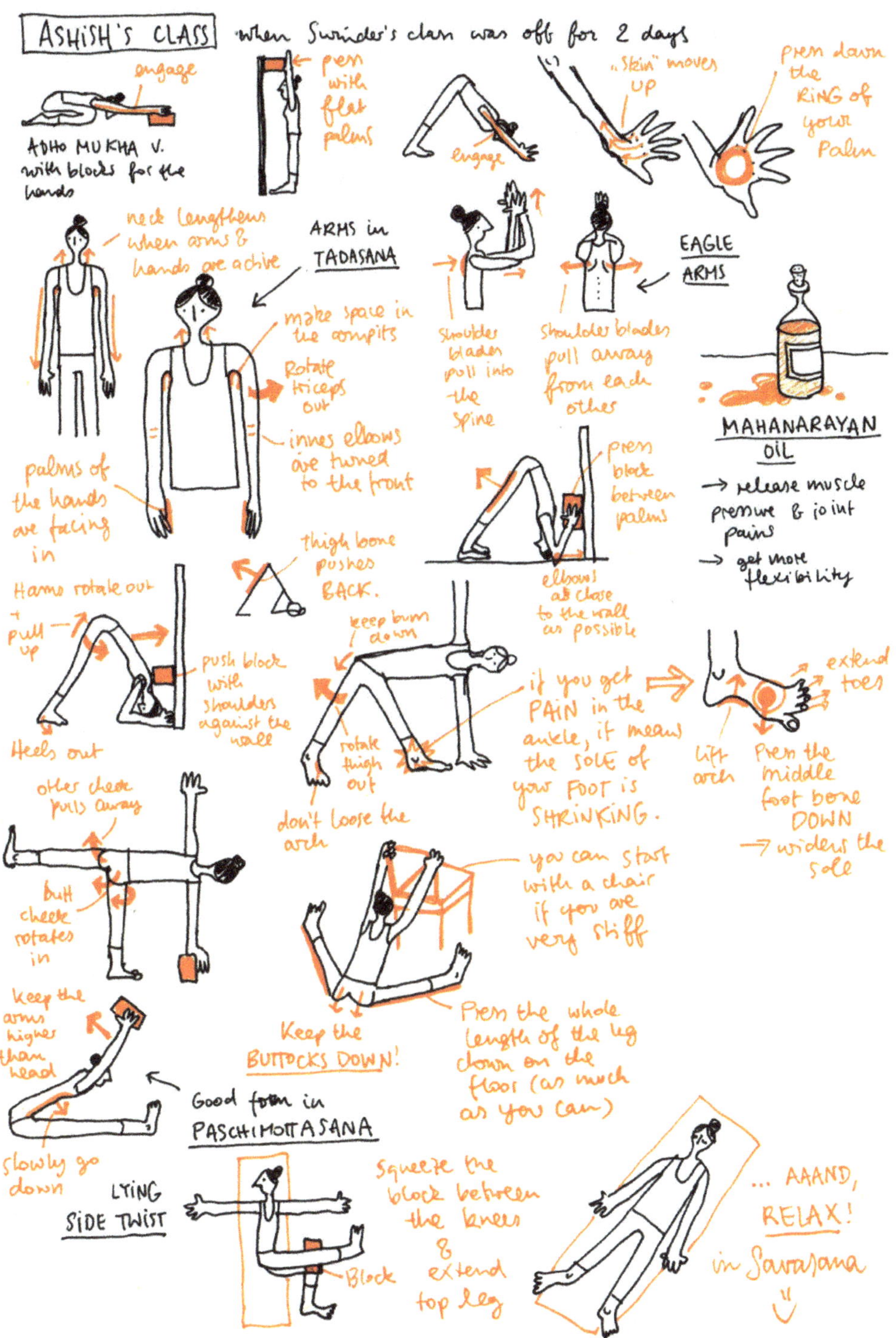

ASHISH'S CLASS
when Swinder's class was off for 2 days
engage
ADHO MUKHA V. with blocks for the hands
press with flat palms
engage
"Skin" moves up
press down the RING of your palm
neck lengthens when arms & hands are active
ARMS in TADASANA
EAGLE ARMS
make space in the armpits
Rotate triceps out
inner elbows are turned to the front
palms of the hands are facing in
shoulder blades pull into the spine
shoulder blades pull away from each other
MAHANARAYAN OIL
→ release muscle pressure & joint pains
→ get more flexibility
thigh bone pushes BACK.
press block between palms
Hams rotate out
pull up
push block with shoulders against the wall
keep bum down
elbows as close to the wall as possible
extend toes
Heels out
rotate thigh out
if you get PAIN in the ankle, it means the SOLE of your FOOT is SHRINKING.
Lift arch
Press the middle foot bone DOWN
→ widens the sole
other cheek pulls away
butt cheek rotates in
don't loose the arch
you can start with a chair if you are very stiff
keep the arms higher than head
Keep the BUTTOCKS DOWN!
Press the whole length of the leg down on the floor (as much as you can)
slowly go down
Good form in PASCHIMOTTASANA
LYING SIDE TWIST
Block
Squeeze the block between the knees & extend top leg
... AAAND, RELAX!
in Savasana

ASHISH'S CLASS | 27 FEB 2017

TADASANA

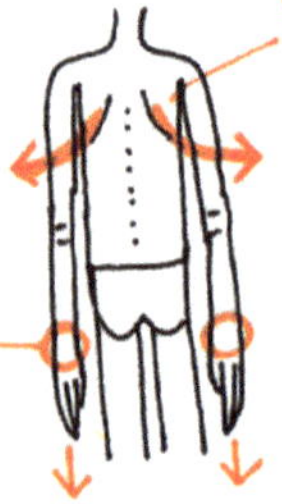

Stretch FINGERS & FOREARMS without HARDENING the WRISTS
↓
this blocks the energy flowing through the arm

Shouldersblades move AWAY from the SPINE and DOWN the BACK & INTO the BODY

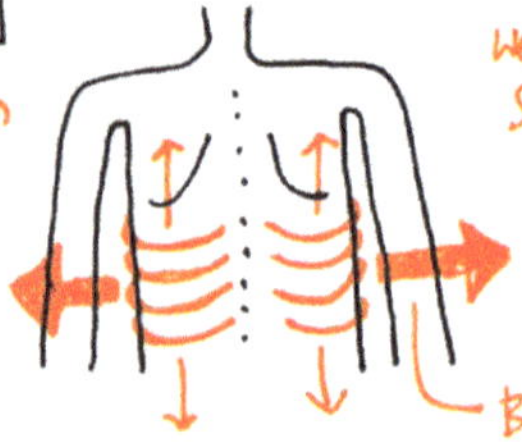

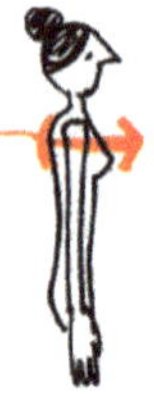

We create SPACE in the SPINE by working with our RIBCAGE.

BROADENING the RIBCAGE & elongating the SIDEBODE automatically STRETCHES the SPINE.

TRIKONASANA

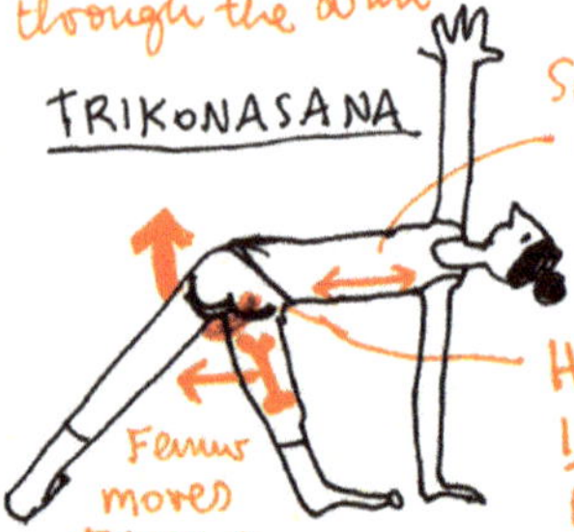

Sidebody LONG

Right Hip rotates IN, then UP to the FRONT.

Femur moves BACK to create SPACE to BEND from the HIP.

ARDHA CHANDRASANA

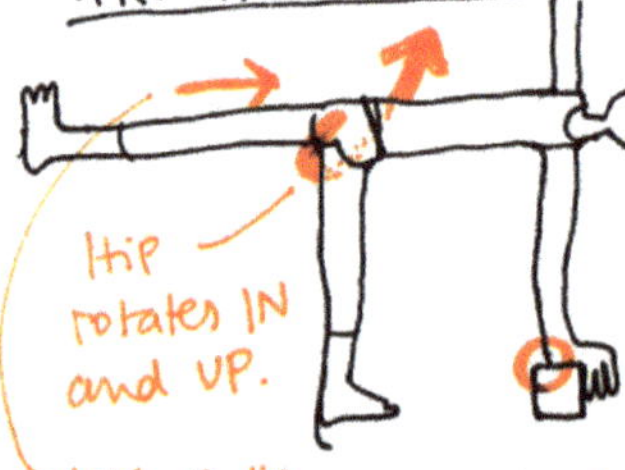

Hip rotates IN and UP.

LEG pulls INTO the HIP.

only press the HEEL of the hand into the BLOCK. Don't HOLD it.

PASHIMOTTANASANA

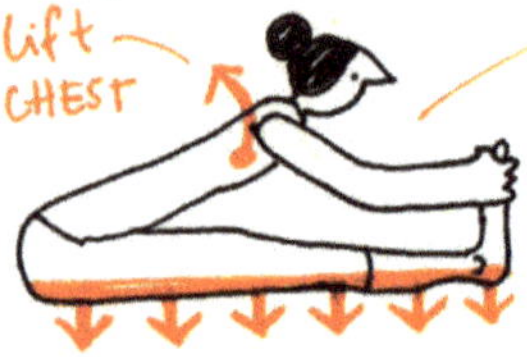

Lift the CHEST

Do A FIRST FOLD (not going fully down) & HOLD it for ~ 10-15 breaths while bringing COMPLETE STILLNESS into the body.

AFTER that, go DEEPER.

PRESSING the LEGS firmly into the ground PROTECTS the LOWER BACK.

RELEASING the LOWER BACK

Hips rotate FORWARD

TRICEPS rotate OUT

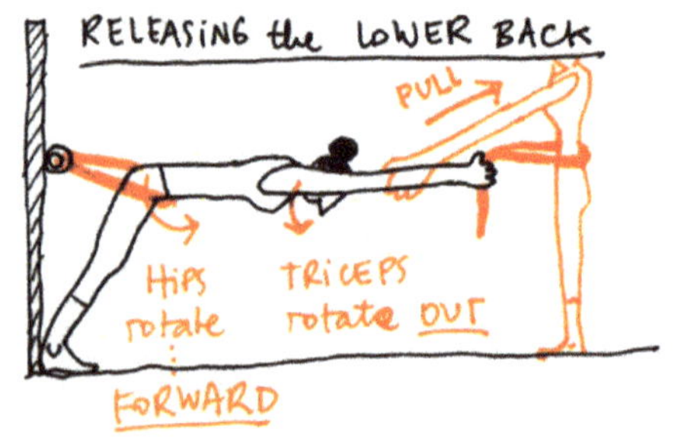

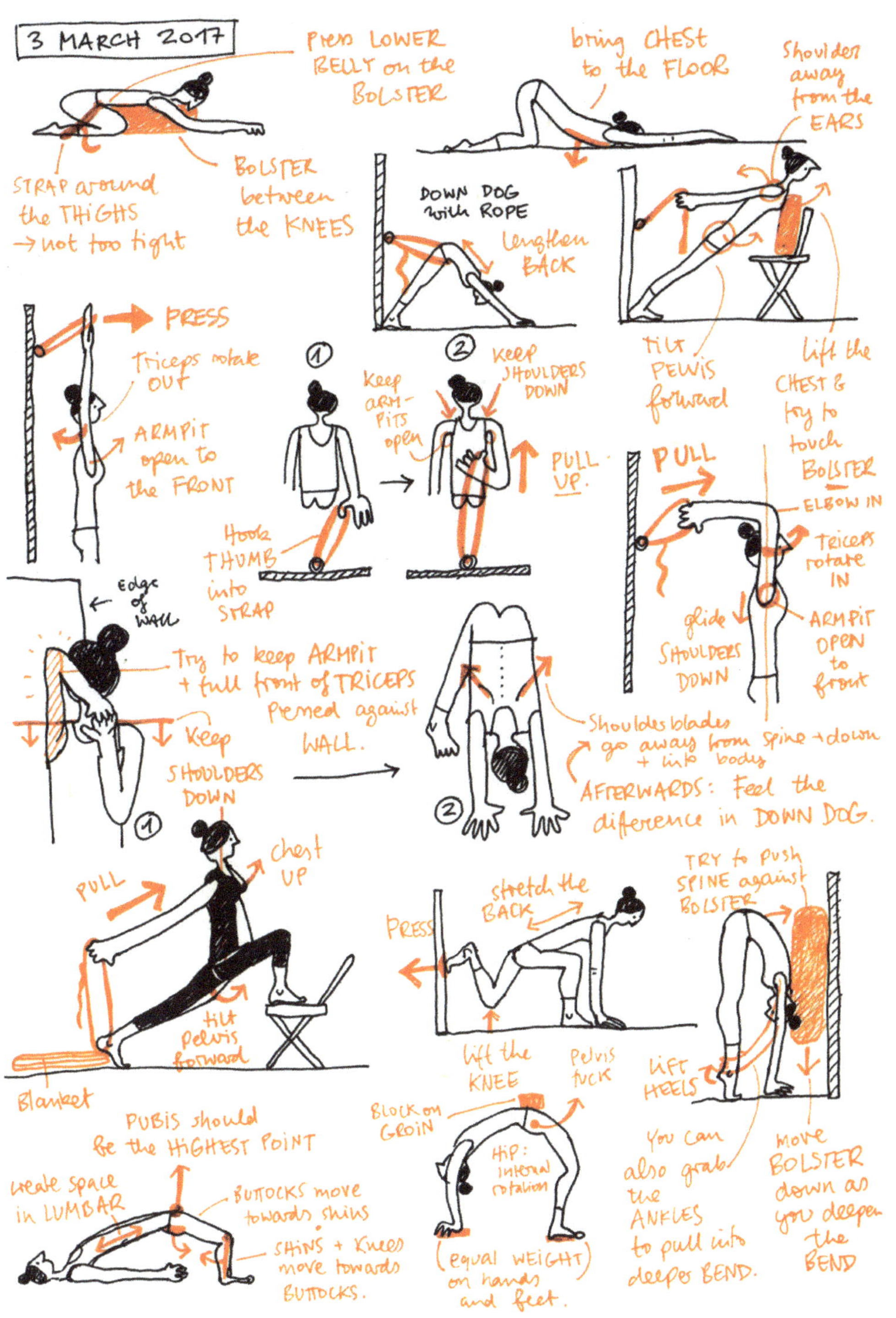

3 MARCH 2017

Press LOWER BELLY on the BOLSTER

bring CHEST to the FLOOR

Shoulder away from the EARS

STRAP around the THIGHS → not too tight

BOLSTER between the KNEES

DOWN DOG with ROPE

Lengthen BACK

PRESS

Triceps rotate OUT

ARMPIT open to the FRONT

① keep ARM-PITS open

Hook THUMB into STRAP

② keep SHOULDERS DOWN

PULL UP.

Tilt PELVIS forward

Lift the CHEST & try to touch BOLSTER

ELBOW IN

Triceps rotate IN

ARMPIT OPEN to front

PULL

glide SHOULDERS DOWN

Edge of WALL

Try to keep ARMPIT + full front of TRICEPS pressed against WALL.

① Keep SHOULDERS DOWN

② Shoulder blades go away from spine + down + into body

AFTERWARDS: Feel the difference in DOWN DOG.

PULL

Chest UP

Press

stretch the BACK

TRY to push SPINE against BOLSTER

tilt pelvis forward

Blanket

lift the KNEE

Pelvis tuck

LIFT HEELS

You can also grab the ANKLES to pull into deeper BEND.

move BOLSTER down as you deepen the BEND

PUBIS should be the HIGHEST POINT

create space in LUMBAR

BUTTOCKS move towards shins

SHINS + KNEES move towards BUTTOCKS.

BLOCK on GROIN

Hip: internal rotation

(equal WEIGHT) on hands and feet.

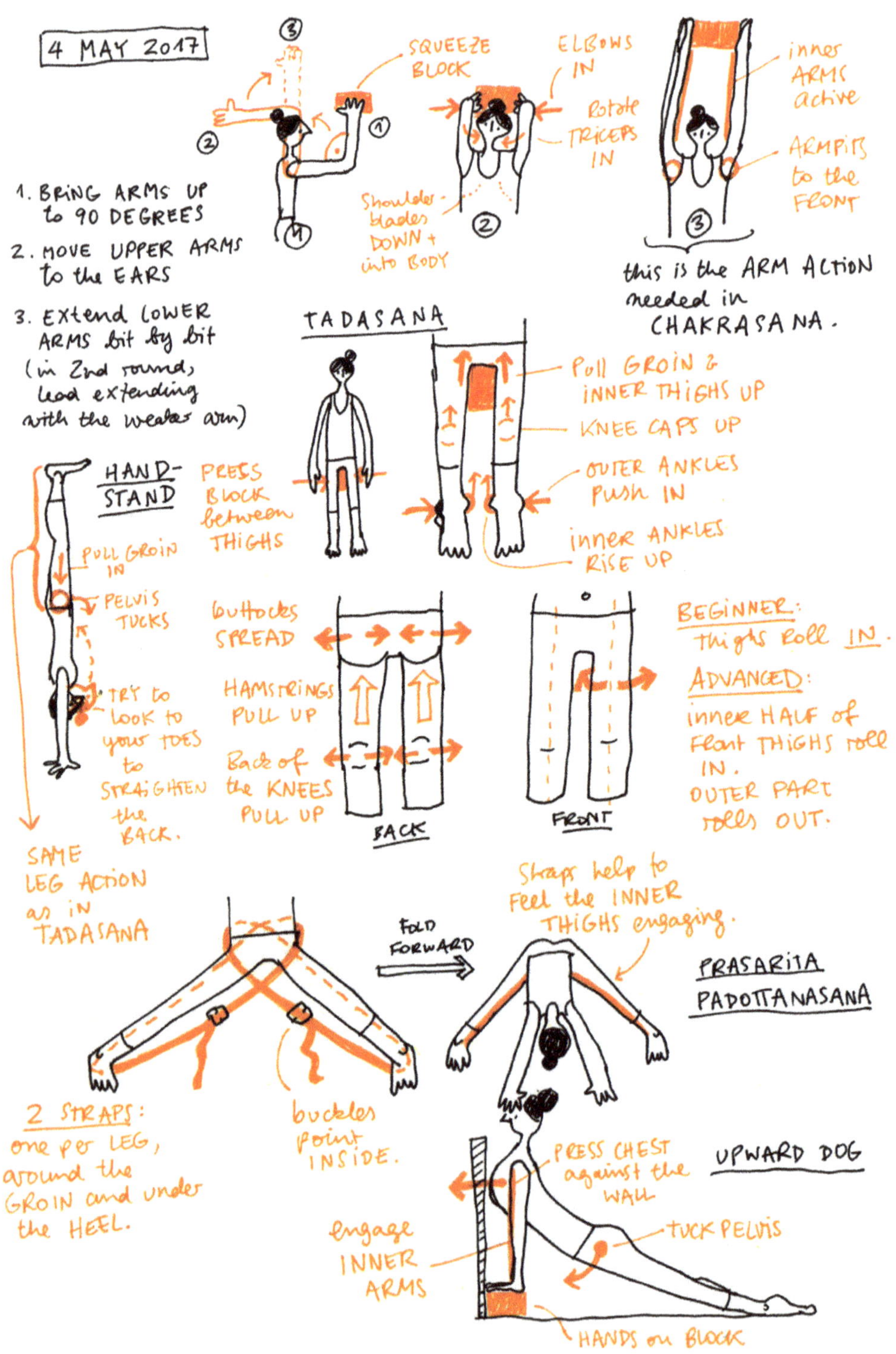

4 MAY 2017

SQUEEZE BLOCK
ELBOWS IN
Rotate TRICEPS IN
inner ARMS active
ARMPITS to the FRONT
Shoulder-blades DOWN + into BODY

this is the ARM ACTION needed in CHAKRASANA.

1. BRING ARMS UP to 90 DEGREES
2. MOVE UPPER ARMS to the EARS
3. Extend LOWER ARMS bit by bit (in 2nd round, lead extending with the weaker arm)

TADASANA

Pull GROIN & INNER THIGHS UP
KNEE CAPS UP
OUTER ANKLES PUSH IN
inner ANKLES RISE UP

HAND-STAND
PRESS BLOCK between THIGHS
PULL GROIN IN
PELVIS TUCKS
TRY to look to your TOES to STRAIGHTEN the BACK.
SAME LEG ACTION as in TADASANA

buttocks SPREAD
HAMSTRINGS PULL UP
Back of the KNEES PULL UP
BACK

FRONT

BEGINNER: thighs roll IN.
ADVANCED: inner HALF of front THIGHS roll IN. OUTER PART rolls OUT.

FOLD FORWARD

Straps help to feel the INNER THIGHS engaging.

PRASARITA PADOTTANASANA

2 STRAPS: one per LEG, around the GROIN and under the HEEL.

buckles point INSIDE.

PRESS CHEST against the WALL

UPWARD DOG

engage INNER ARMS

TUCK PELVIS

HANDS on BLOCK

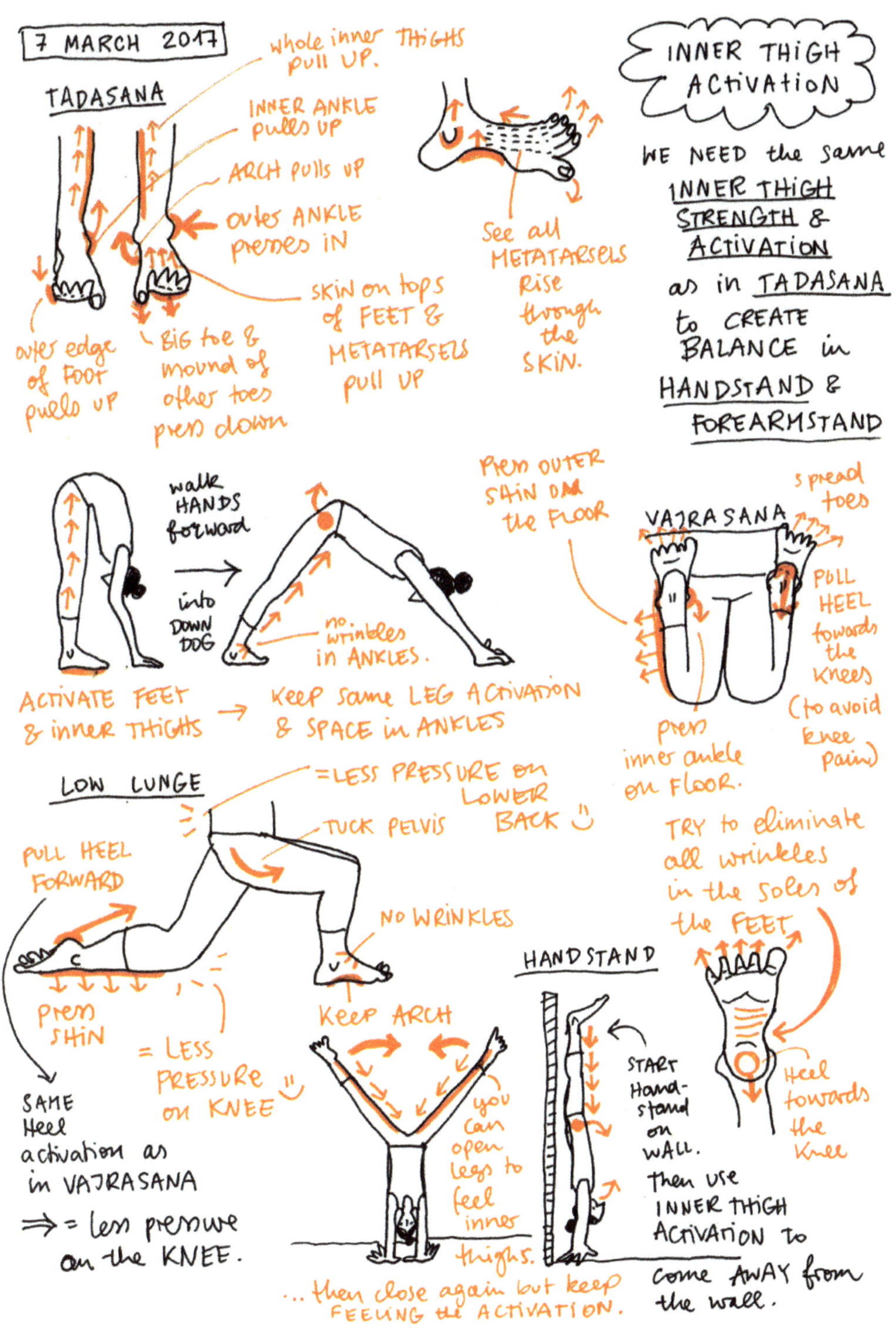

7 MARCH 2017
TADASANA
whole inner THIGHS pull UP.
INNER ANKLE pulls UP
ARCH pulls UP
outer ANKLE presses IN
Skin on tops of FEET & METATARSELS pull UP
outer edge of FOOT pulls UP
Big toe & mound of other toes press down
See all METATARSELS Rise through the SKIN.
INNER THIGH ACTIVATION
WE NEED the same INNER THIGH STRENGTH & ACTIVATION as in TADASANA to CREATE BALANCE in HANDSTAND & FOREARMSTAND
walk HANDS forward into DOWN DOG
ACTIVATE FEET & inner THIGHS
Press OUTER SHIN on the FLOOR
no wrinkles in ANKLES.
KEEP same LEG ACTIVATION & SPACE in ANKLES
VAJRASANA
spread toes
PULL HEEL towards the knees (to avoid knee pain)
Press inner ankle on FLOOR.
LOW LUNGE
PULL HEEL FORWARD
= LESS PRESSURE on LOWER BACK
TUCK PELVIS
NO WRINKLES
Press SHIN
= LESS PRESSURE on KNEE
KEEP ARCH
SAME Heel activation as in VAJRASANA
⇒ = less pressure on the KNEE.
you can open legs to feel inner thighs.
...then close again but keep FEELING the ACTIVATION.
HANDSTAND
START Hand-stand on WALL.
then use INNER THIGH ACTIVATION to come AWAY from the wall.
TRY to eliminate all wrinkles in the soles of the FEET
Heel towards the knee

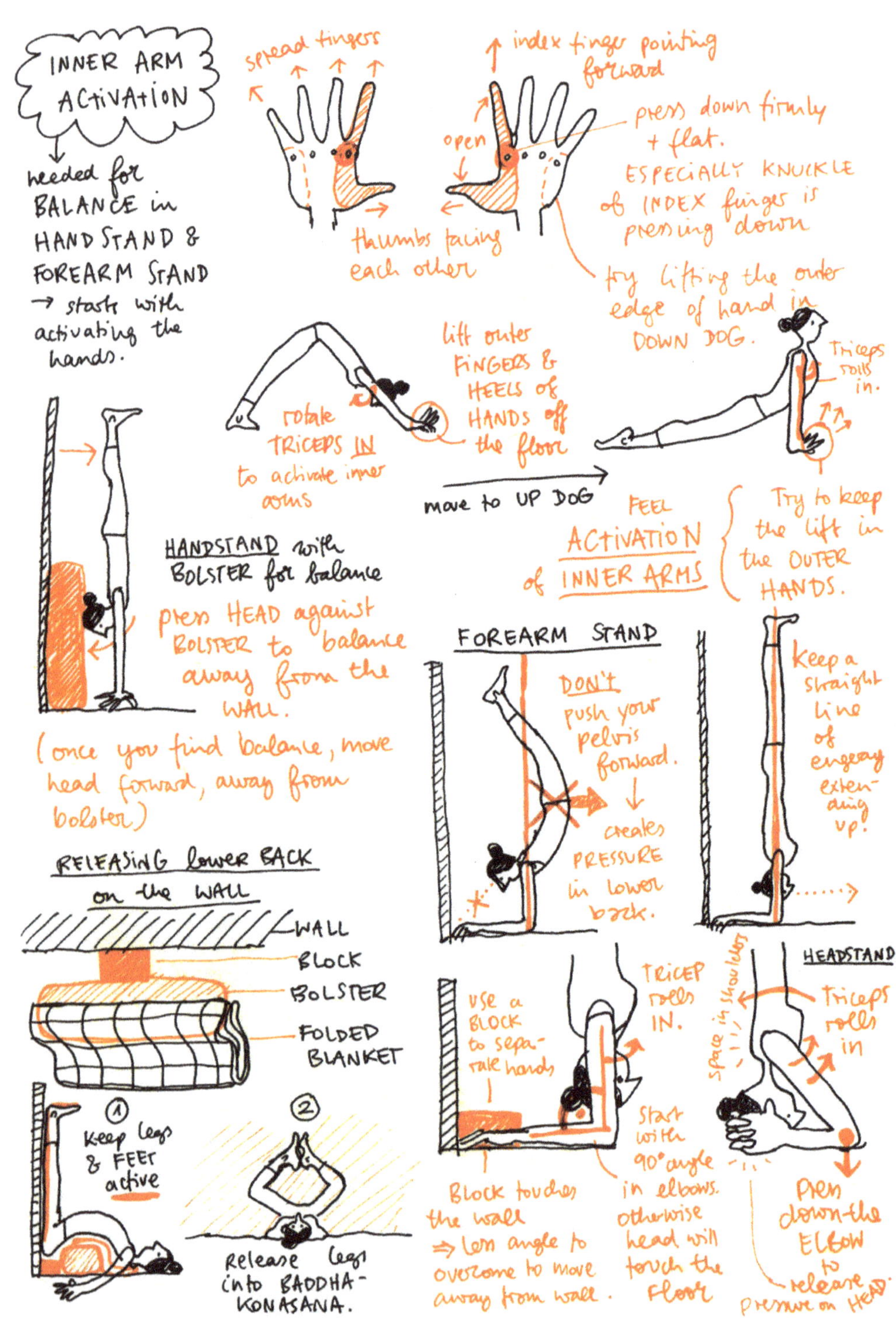

INNER ARM ACTIVATION

needed for BALANCE in HAND STAND & FOREARM STAND
→ start with activating the hands.

spread fingers
thumbs facing each other

index finger pointing forward
open
press down firmly + flat. ESPECIALLY KNUCKLE of INDEX finger is pressing down
try lifting the outer edge of hand in DOWN DOG.
Triceps rolls in.

rotate TRICEPS IN to activate inner arms
lift outer FINGERS & HEELS of HANDS off the floor
move to UP DOG
FEEL ACTIVATION of INNER ARMS
Try to keep the lift in the OUTER HANDS.

HANDSTAND with BOLSTER for balance
press HEAD against BOLSTER to balance away from the WALL.
(once you find balance, move head forward, away from bolster)

FOREARM STAND
DON'T push your pelvis forward.
↓ creates PRESSURE in lower back.
Keep a straight line of energy extending up!

RELEASING lower BACK on the WALL
WALL
BLOCK
BOLSTER
FOLDED BLANKET
① keep legs & FEET active
② Release legs into BADDHA-KONASANA.

USE a BLOCK to separate hands
TRICEP rolls IN.
Start with 90° angle in elbows. otherwise head will touch the floor
Block touches the wall → less angle to overcome to move away from wall.

HEADSTAND
space in shoulders
Triceps rolls in
Press down the ELBOW to release pressure on HEAD

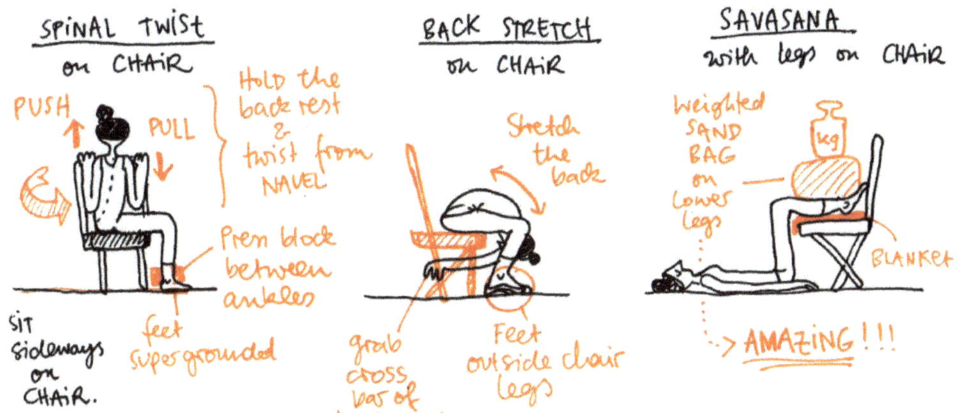

SPINAL TWIST
on CHAIR
PUSH
PULL
Hold the back rest & twist from NAVEL
Press block between ankles
Sit sideways on CHAIR.
feet super grounded
BACK STRETCH
on CHAIR
Stretch the back
grab cross bar of back legs
Feet outside chair legs
SAVASANA
with legs on CHAIR
Weighted SAND BAG on lower legs
kg
BLANKet
AMAZING!!!

ANATOMY

TAUGHT BY
GURMEET SINGH

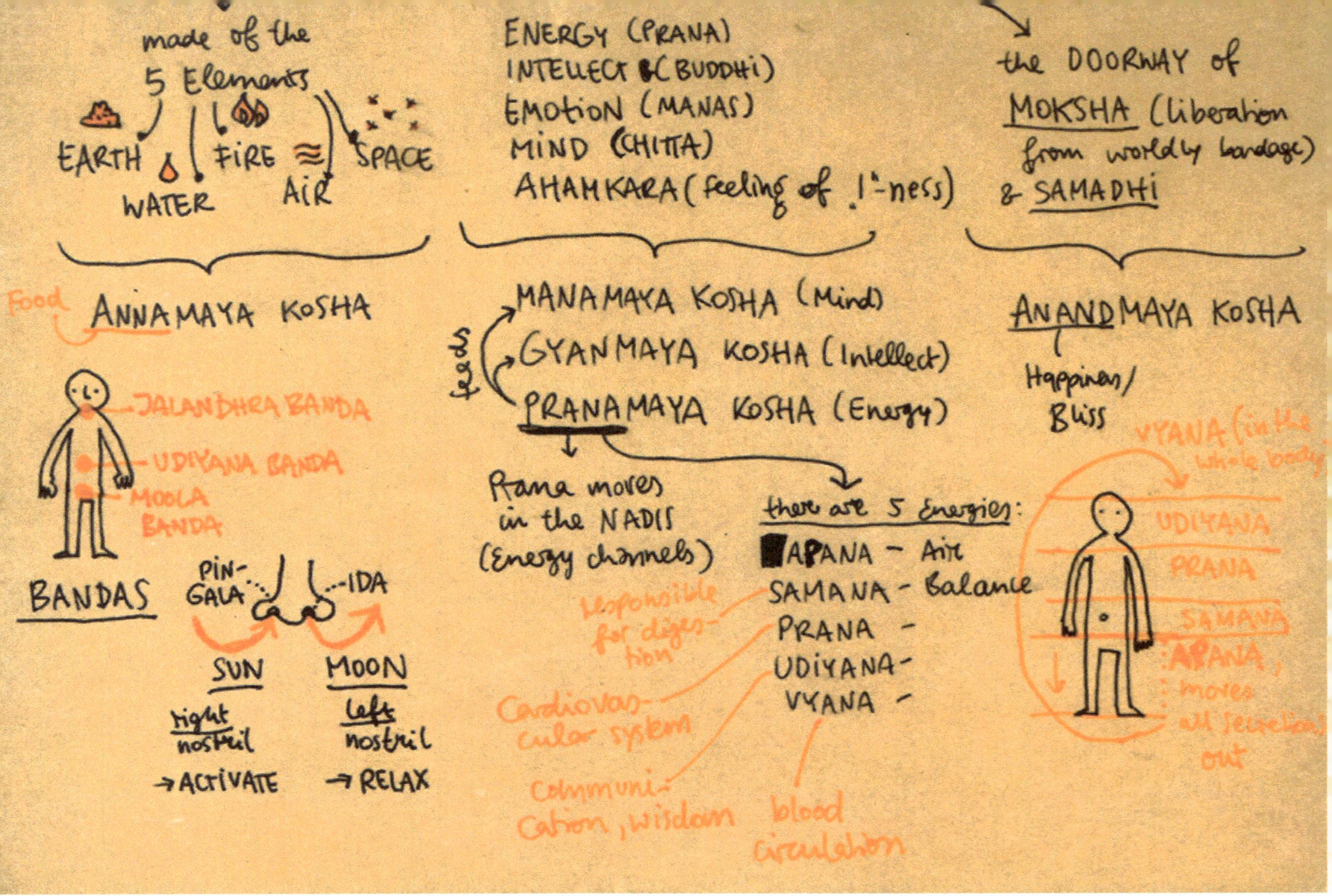

made of the
5 Elements

EARTH
WATER
FIRE
AIR
SPACE

ENERGY (PRANA)
INTELLECT & (BUDDHI)
EMOTION (MANAS)
MIND (CHITTA)
AHAMKARA (feeling of "I"-ness)

the DOORWAY of
MOKSHA (liberation from worldly bondage)
& SAMADHI

Food
ANNAMAYA KOSHA

MANAMAYA KOSHA (Mind)
feeds → GYANMAYA KOSHA (Intellect)
PRANAMAYA KOSHA (Energy)

ANANDMAYA KOSHA

Happiness/
Bliss

JALANDHRA BANDA
UDIYANA BANDA
MOOLA BANDA

BANDAS

PIN-GALA
IDA
SUN
right nostril
→ ACTIVATE
MOON
left nostril
→ RELAX

Prana moves
in the NADIS
(Energy channels)

there are 5 Energies:
APANA — Air
SAMANA — Balance
PRANA —
UDIYANA —
VYANA —

responsible for digestion
Cardiovascular system
communication, wisdom
blood circulation

VYANA (in the whole body)
UDIYANA
PRANA
SAMANA
APANA, moves all secretions out

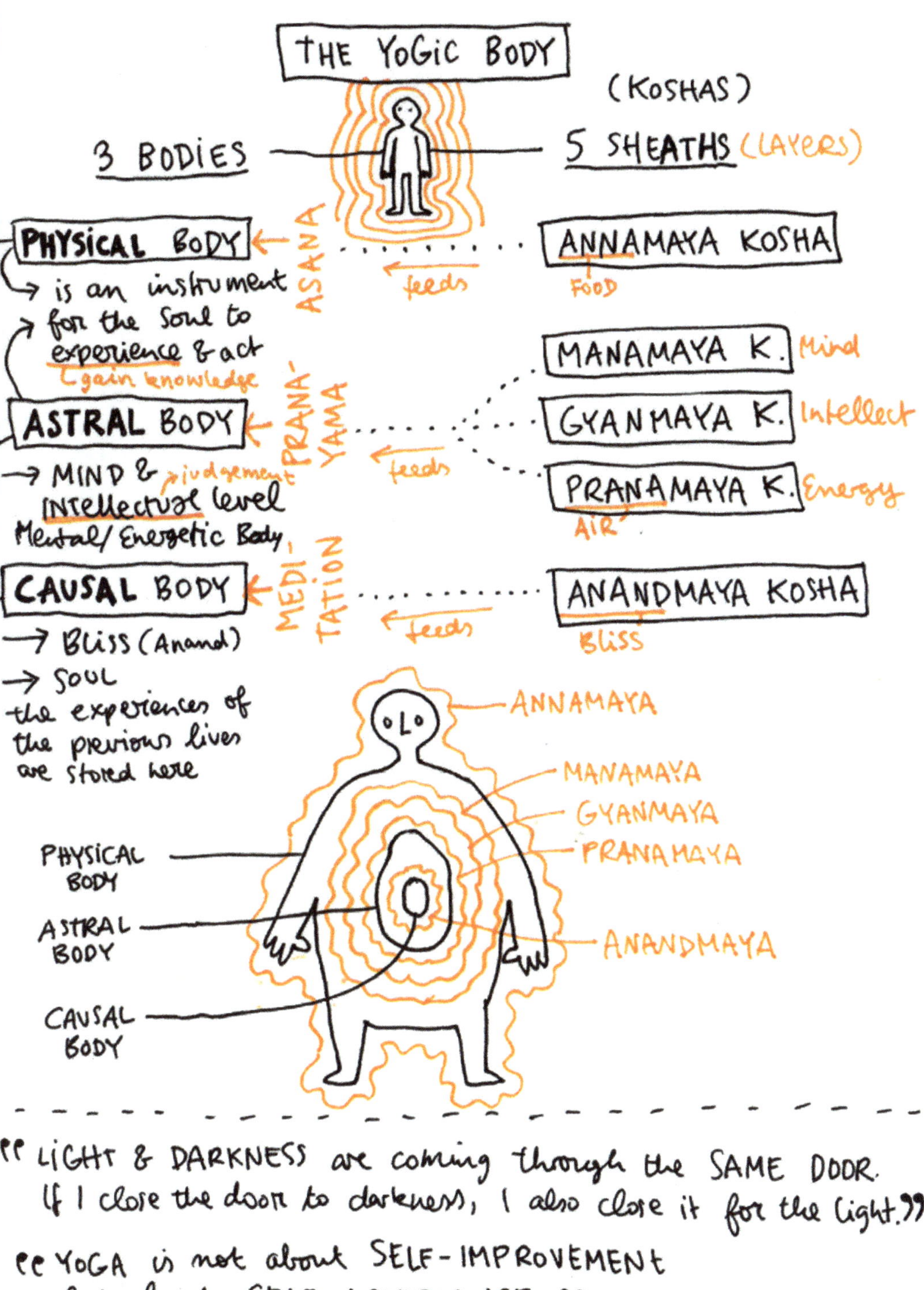

" LIGHT & DARKNESS are coming through the SAME DOOR. If I close the door to darkness, I also close it for the light. "

" YOGA is not about SELF-IMPROVEMENT but about SELF-ACCEPTANCE. "

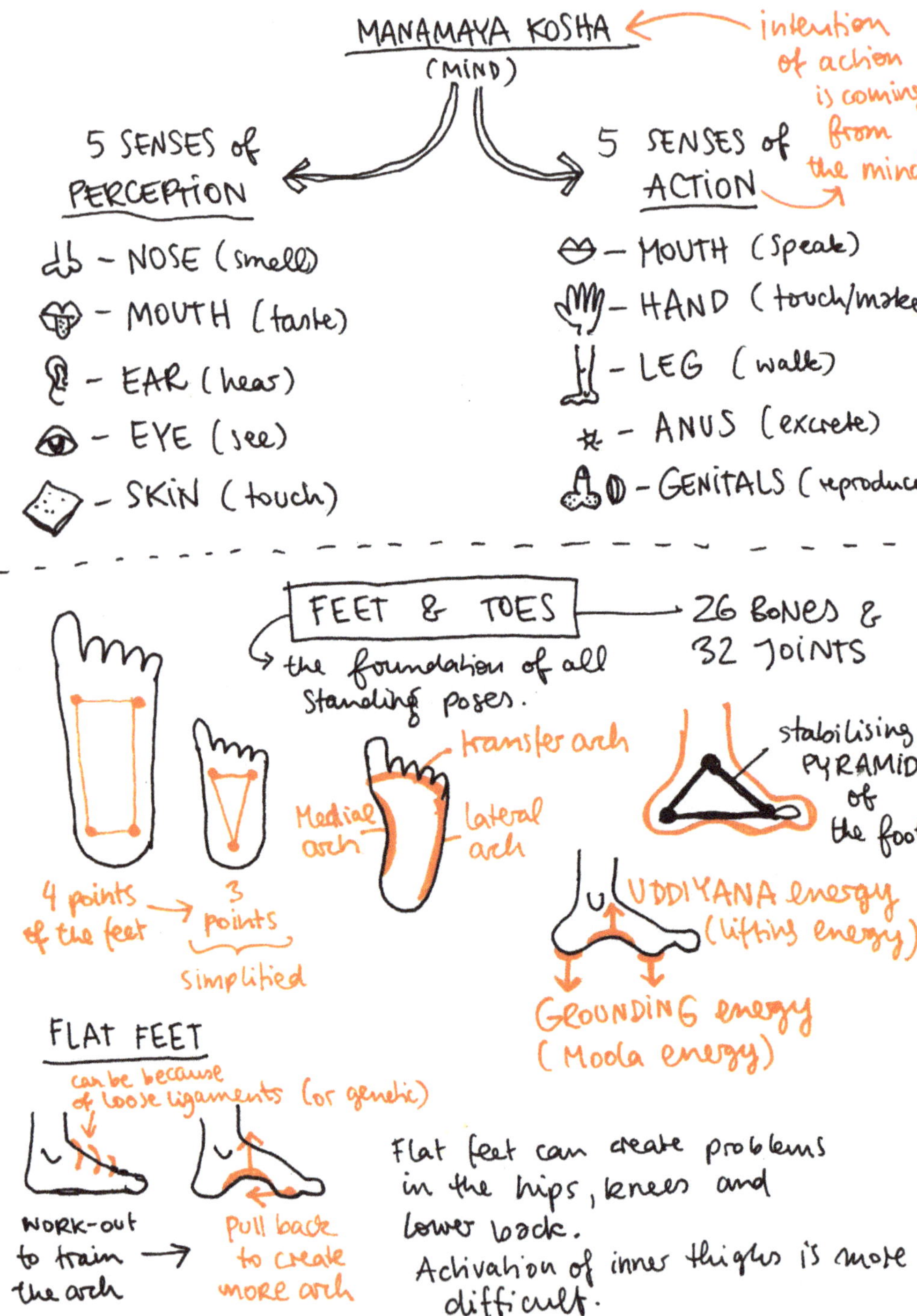

MANAMAYA KOSHA
(MIND)
intention of action is coming from the mind
5 SENSES of PERCEPTION
- NOSE (smell)
- MOUTH (taste)
- EAR (hear)
- EYE (see)
- SKIN (touch)
5 SENSES of ACTION
- MOUTH (speak)
- HAND (touch/make)
- LEG (walk)
- ANUS (excrete)
- GENITALS (reproduce)
FEET & TOES
the foundation of all standing poses.
26 BONES & 32 JOINTS
transfer arch
Medial arch
lateral arch
stabilising PYRAMID of the foot
4 points of the feet
3 points
simplified
UDDIYANA energy (lifting energy)
GROUNDING energy (Moola energy)
FLAT FEET
can be because of loose ligaments (or genetic)
WORK-OUT to train the arch
Pull back to create more arch
Flat feet can create problems in the hips, knees and lower back.
Activation of inner thighs is more difficult.

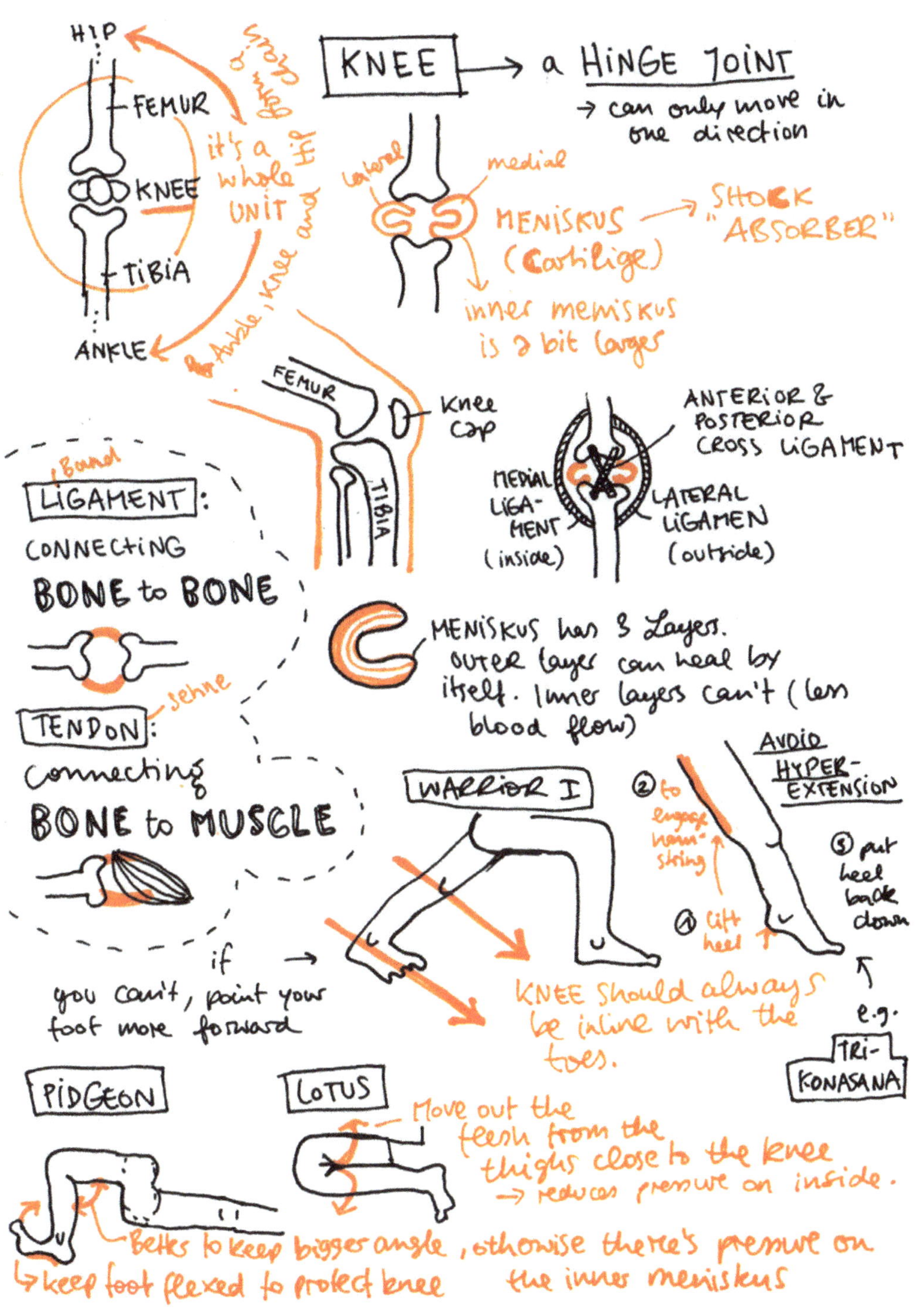

HIP
FEMUR
KNEE
TIBIA
ANKLE
it's a whole UNIT
it's all connected
→ Ankle, knee and Hip

KNEE → a HINGE JOINT
→ can only move in one direction

lateral   medial
MENISKUS (Cartilige) → SHOCK "ABSORBER"
inner meniskus is a bit larger

FEMUR
Knee Cap
TIBIA

ANTERIOR & POSTERIOR CROSS LIGAMENT
MEDIAL LIGA- MENT (inside)
LATERAL LIGAMEN (outside)

LIGAMENT: Band
CONNECTING BONE to BONE

MENISKUS has 3 Layers. outer layer can heal by itself. Inner layers can't (less blood flow)

TENDON: Sehne
Connecting BONE to MUSCLE

if → you can't, point your foot more forward

WARRIOR I
② to engage ham-string
① Lift heel
KNEE should always be inline with the toes.

AVOID HYPER-EXTENSION
③ put heel back down
e.g.
TRI-KONASANA

PIDGEON
→ keep foot flexed to protect knee

LOTUS
Move out the flesh from the thighs close to the knee → reduces pressure on inside.
Better to keep bigger angle, otherwise there's pressure on the inner meniskus

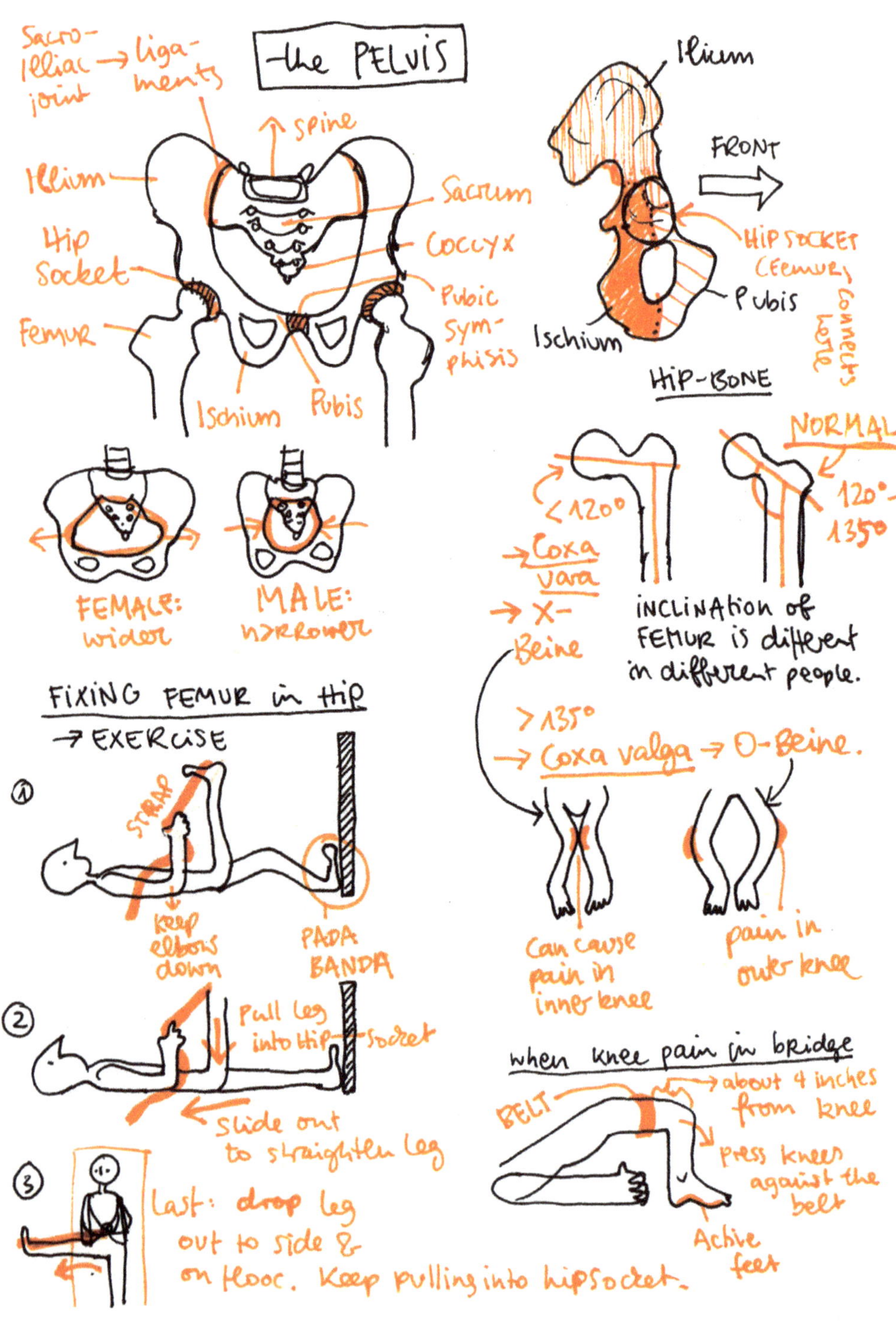
the PELVIS

Sacro-Iliac joint → liga-ments
Ilium
Hip Socket
Femur
spine
Sacrum
Coccyx
Pubic Symphisis
Ischium
Pubis

Ilium
FRONT
HIP SOCKET (FEMUR) connects here
Pubis
Ischium
HIP-BONE

FEMALE: wider
MALE: narrower

NORMAL
120° - 135°
< 120°
Coxa vara
→ X-Beine
> 135°
→ Coxa valga → O-Beine.
INCLINATION of FEMUR is different in different people.
Can cause pain in inner knee
pain in outer knee

FIXING FEMUR in hip
→ EXERCISE
① STRAP
keep elbows down
PADA BANDA
② Pull leg into hip socket
slide out to straighten leg
③ Last: drop leg out to side & on floor. Keep pulling into hip socket.

when knee pain in bridge
BELT
→ about 4 inches from knee
press knees against the belt
Active feet

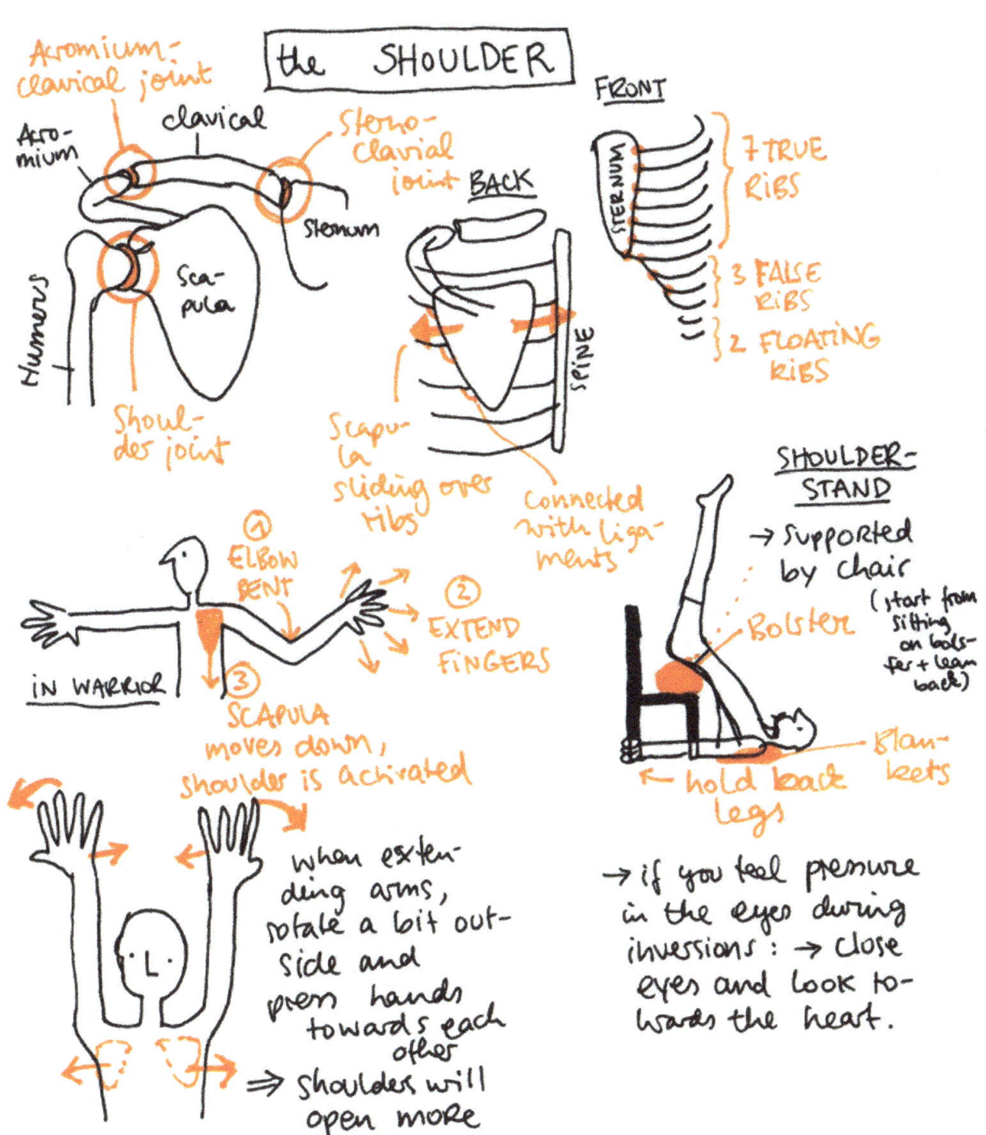

the SHOULDER
FRONT
Acromium-clavical joint
Acromium
clavical
Sterno-clavical joint
BACK
Sternum
Sca-pula
Humerus
Shoulder joint
STERNUM
7 TRUE RIBS
3 FALSE RIBS
2 FLOATING RIBS
SPINE
Scapula sliding over ribs
connected with ligaments
SHOULDER-STAND
→ supported by chair
(start from sitting on bolster + lean back)
Bolster
Blankets
← hold back legs
① ELBOW BENT
② EXTEND FINGERS
③ SCAPULA moves down, shoulder is activated
IN WARRIOR
L
when extending arms, rotate a bit outside and press hands towards each other
⇒ shoulders will open more
→ if you feel pressure in the eyes during inversions: → close eyes and look towards the heart.

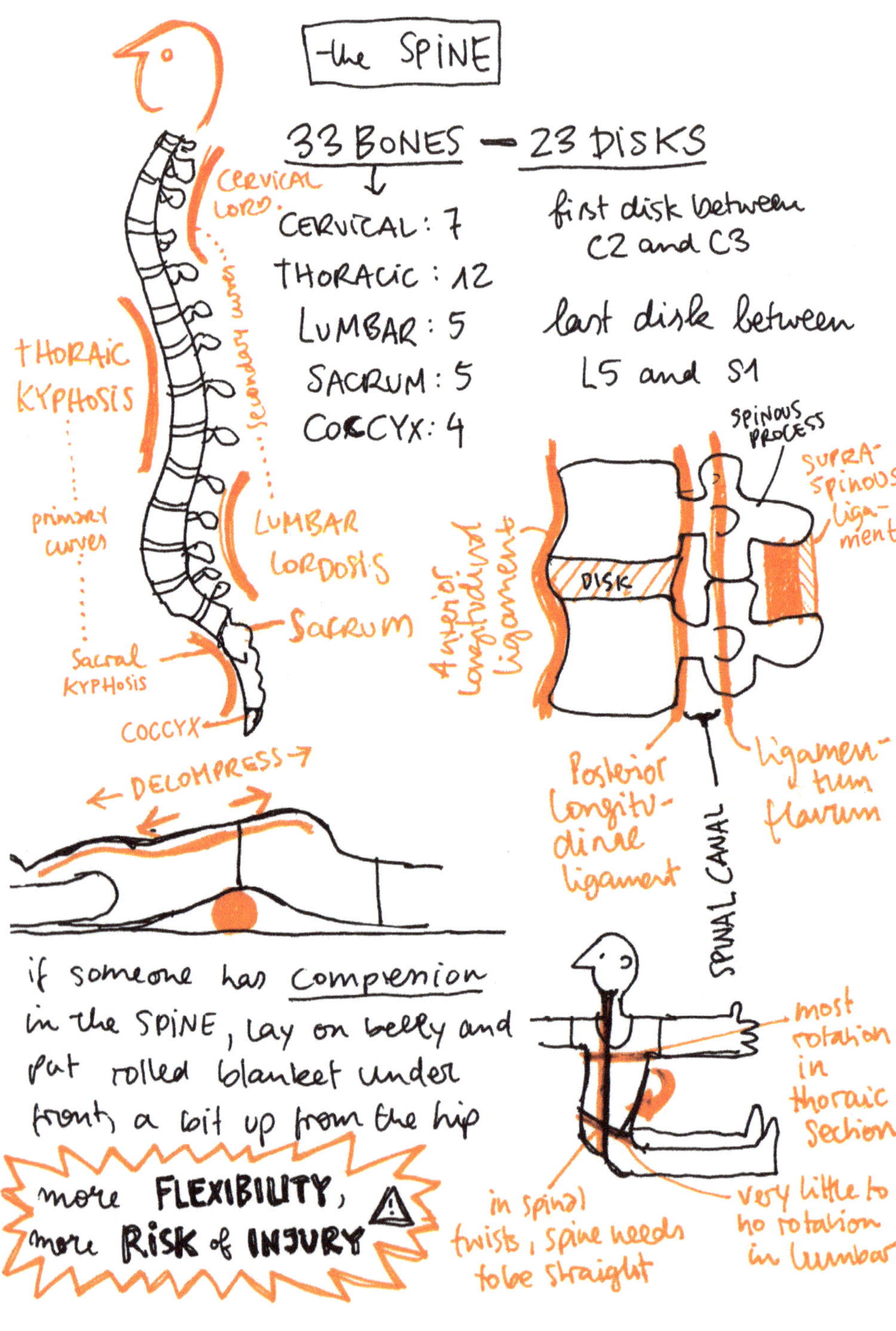

the SPINE

33 BONES — 23 DISKS

CERVICAL: 7
THORACIC: 12
LUMBAR: 5
SACRUM: 5
COCCYX: 4

first disk between C2 and C3

last disk between L5 and S1

CERVICAL LORD.
THORACIC KYPHOSIS
secondary curves
primary curves
LUMBAR LORDOSIS
Sacrum
Sacral KYPHOSIS
COCCYX

SPINOUS PROCESS
SUPRA-SPINOUS liga-ment
Anterior Longitudinal ligament
DISK
Posterior Longitu-dinal ligament
SPINAL CANAL
Ligamen-tum flavum

DECOMPRESS

if someone has compression in the SPINE, lay on belly and put rolled blanket under front, a bit up from the hip

more FLEXIBILITY, more RISK of INJURY

most rotation in thoracic section
very little to no rotation in lumbar
in spinal twists, spine needs to be straight

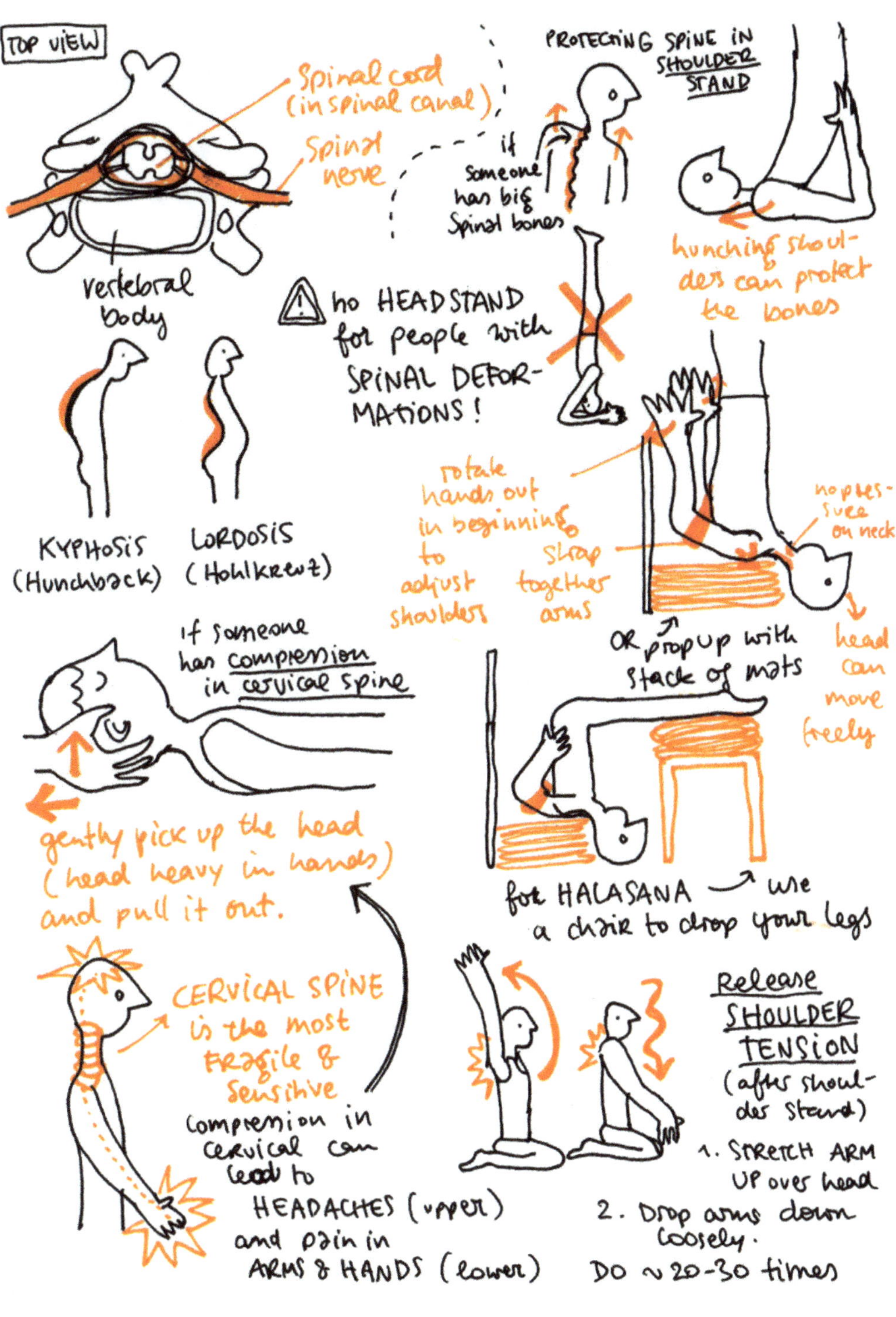

TOP VIEW
Spinal cord (in spinal canal)
Spinal nerve
vertebral body
KYPHOSIS (Hunchback)
LORDOSIS (Hohlkreuz)
if someone has big spinal bones
no HEADSTAND for people with SPINAL DEFORMATIONS !
PROTECTING SPINE IN SHOULDER STAND
hunching shoulders can protect the bones
rotate hands out in beginning to adjust shoulders
strap together arms
OR prop up with stack of mats
no pressure on neck
head can move freely
if someone has compression in cervical spine
gently pick up the head (head heavy in hands) and pull it out.
for HALASANA → use a chair to drop your legs
CERVICAL SPINE is the most fragile & sensitive
compression in cervical can lead to HEADACHES (upper) and pain in ARMS & HANDS (lower)
Release SHOULDER TENSION (after shoulder stand)
1. STRETCH ARM UP over head
2. Drop arms down loosely.
DO ~ 20-30 times

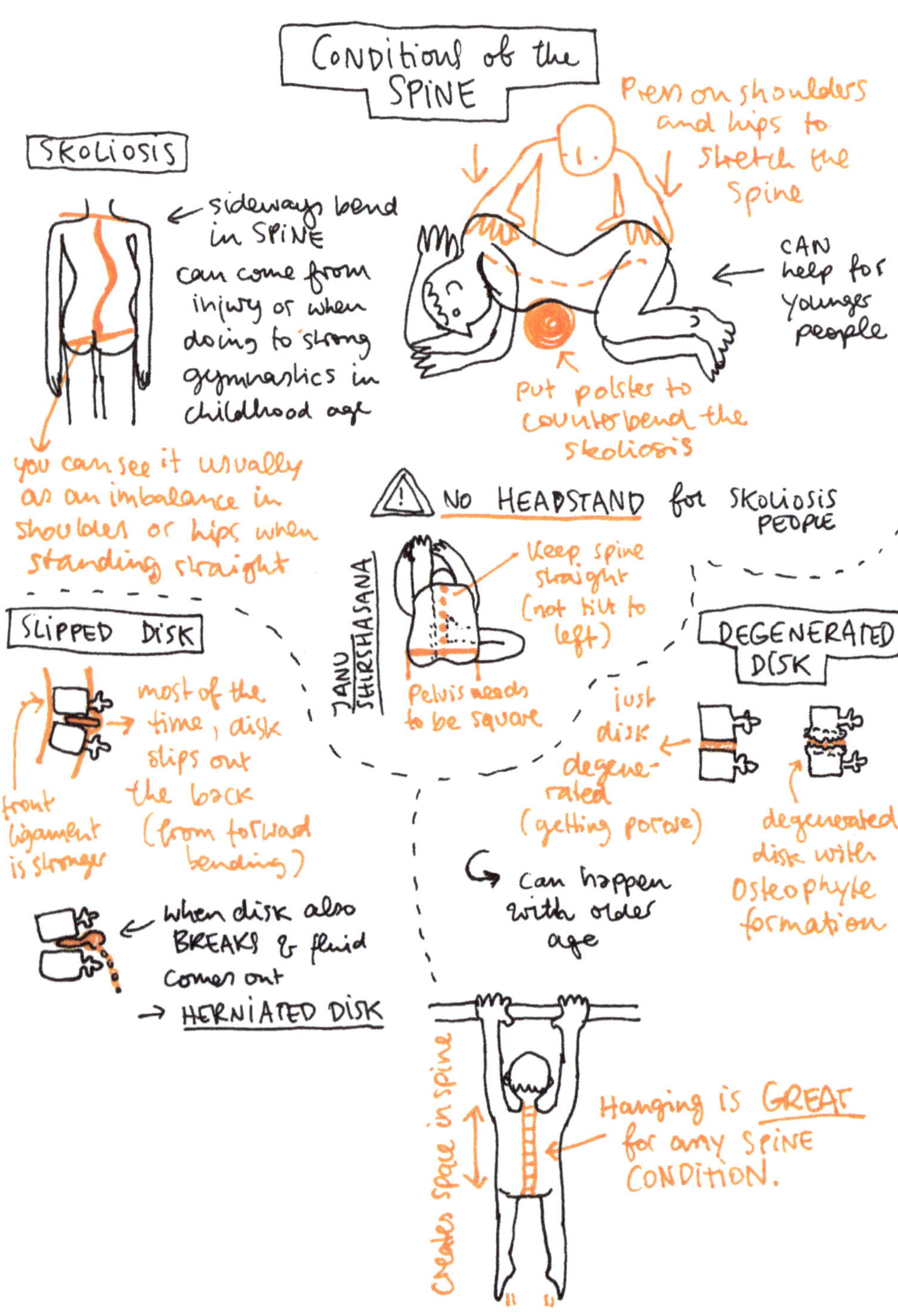

Conditions of the SPINE

SKOLIOSIS

← sideways bend in SPINE
can come from injury or when doing to strong gymnastics in childhood age

you can see it usually as an imbalance in shoulders or hips when standing straight

Press on shoulders and hips to stretch the spine

CAN help for younger people

put polster to counterbend the skoliosis

⚠ NO HEADSTAND for SKOLIOSIS PEOPLE

JANU SHIRSHASANA
Keep spine straight (not tilt to left)
Pelvis needs to be square

SLIPPED DISK

most of the time, disk slips out the back (from forward bending)
front ligament is stronger

when disk also BREAKS & fluid comes out
→ HERNIATED DISK

DEGENERATED DISK

just disk degenerated (getting porose)
can happen with older age
degenerated disk with osteophyte formation

Creates space in spine
Hanging is GREAT for any spine CONDITION.

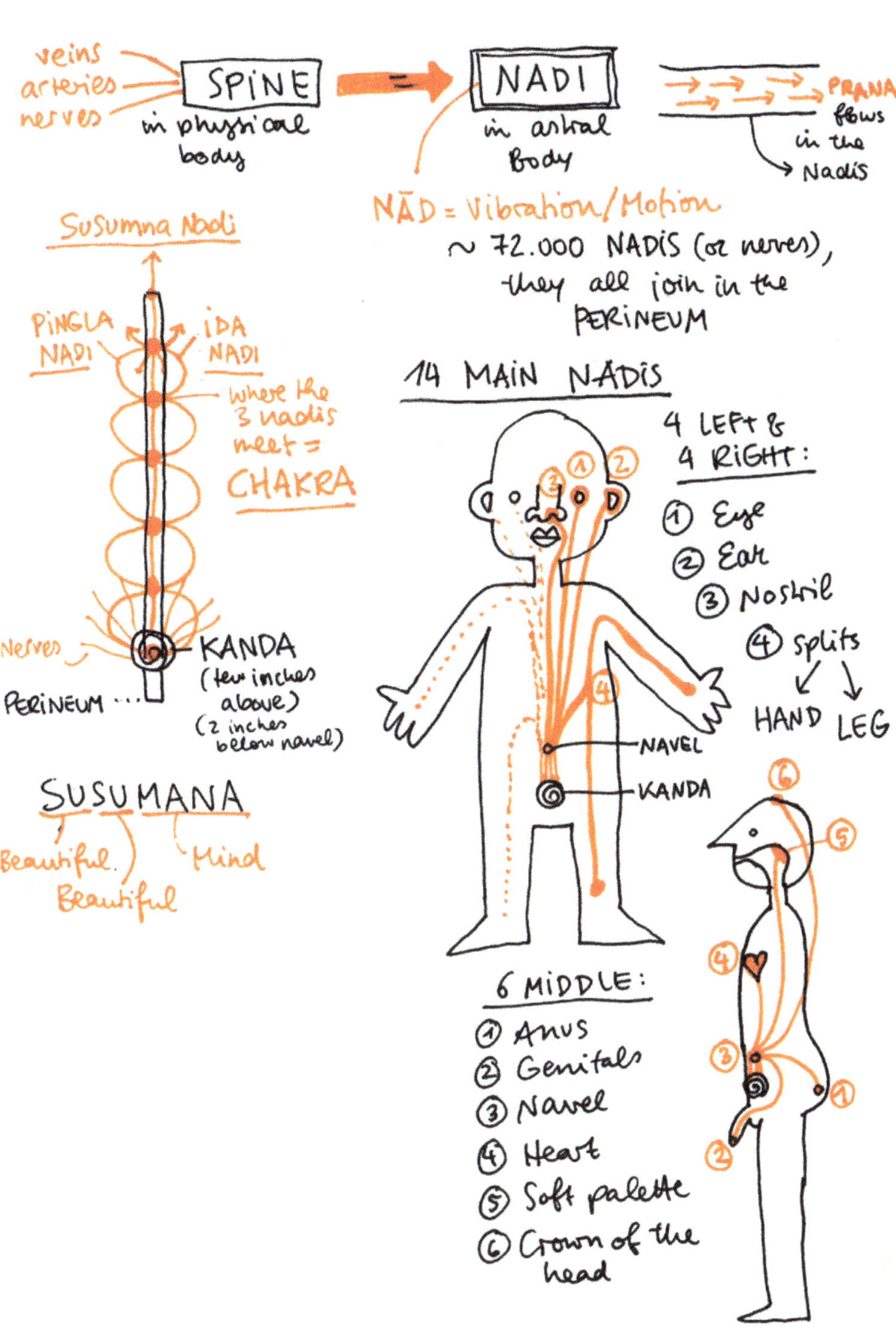

veins
arteries
nerves
SPINE
in physical body
=
NADI
in astral Body
PRANA flows in the Nadis

NĀD = Vibration/Motion
~ 72.000 NADIS (or nerves), they all join in the PERINEUM

Susumna Nadi
PINGLA NADI
IDA NADI
where the 3 nadis meet = CHAKRA
Nerves
PERINEUM ...
KANDA (few inches above) (2 inches below navel)

SUSUMANA
Beautiful
Beautiful
Mind

14 MAIN NADIS
4 LEFT & 4 RIGHT:
① Eye
② Ear
③ Nostril
④ splits
HAND   LEG
NAVEL
KANDA

6 MIDDLE:
① Anus
② Genitals
③ Navel
④ Heart
⑤ Soft palette
⑥ Crown of the head

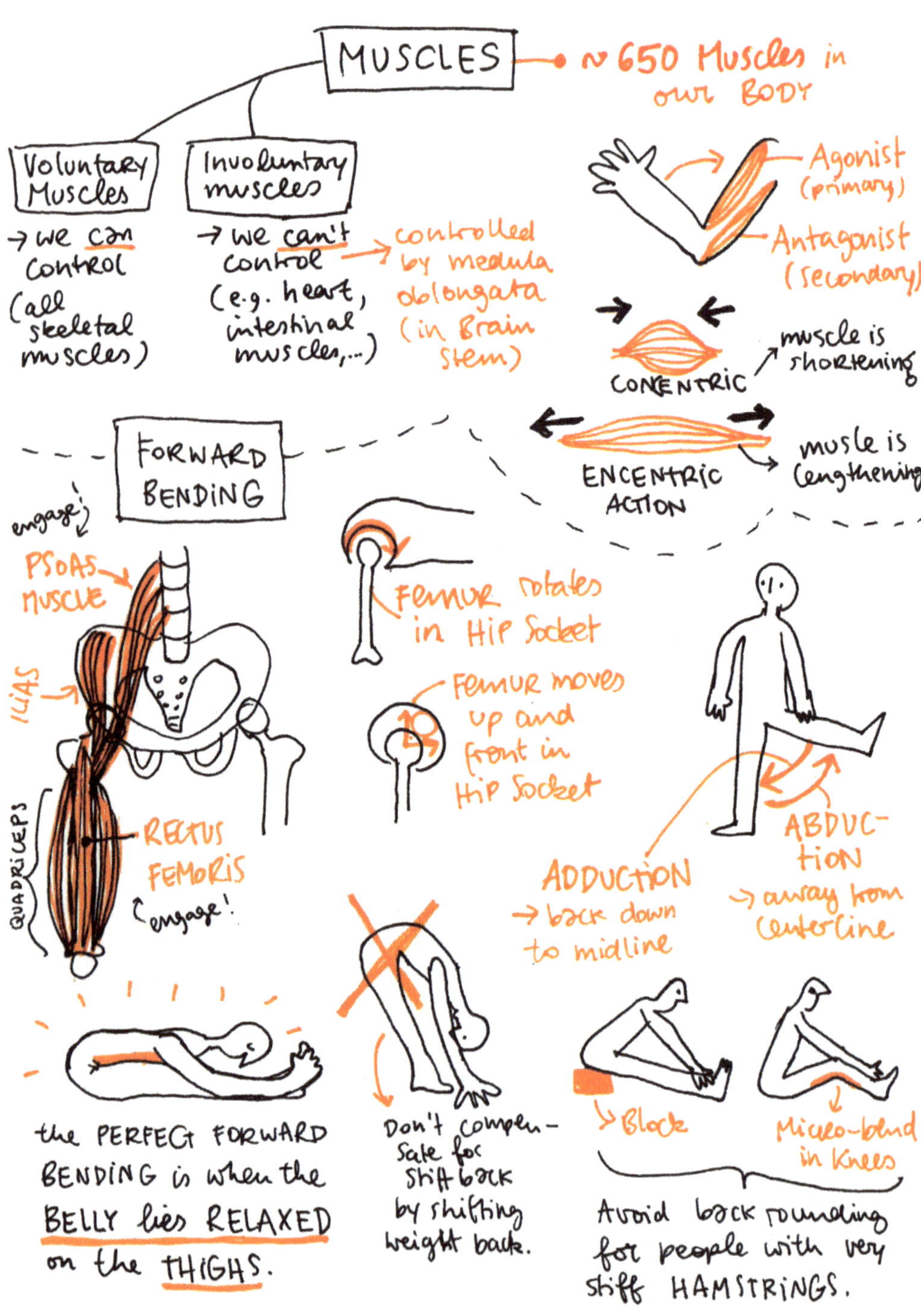

MUSCLES
~ 650 Muscles in our BODY

Voluntary Muscles
→ we can control (all skeletal muscles)

Involuntary muscles
→ we can't control (e.g. heart, intestinal muscles,...)
controlled by medulla oblongata (in Brain stem)

Agonist (primary)
Antagonist (secondary)

CONCENTRIC
muscle is shortening

ENCENTRIC ACTION
musle is lengthening

FORWARD BENDING

engage!
PSOAS MUSCLE
ILIAS
QUADRICEPS
RECTUS FEMORIS
engage!

Femur rotates in Hip Socket
Femur moves up and front in Hip Socket

ADDUCTION
→ back down to midline

ABDUCTION
→ away from center line

the PERFECT FORWARD BENDING is when the BELLY lies RELAXED on the THIGHS.

Don't compensate for stiff back by shifting weight back.

→ Block
Micro-bend in Knees

Avoid back rounding for people with very stiff HAMSTRINGS.

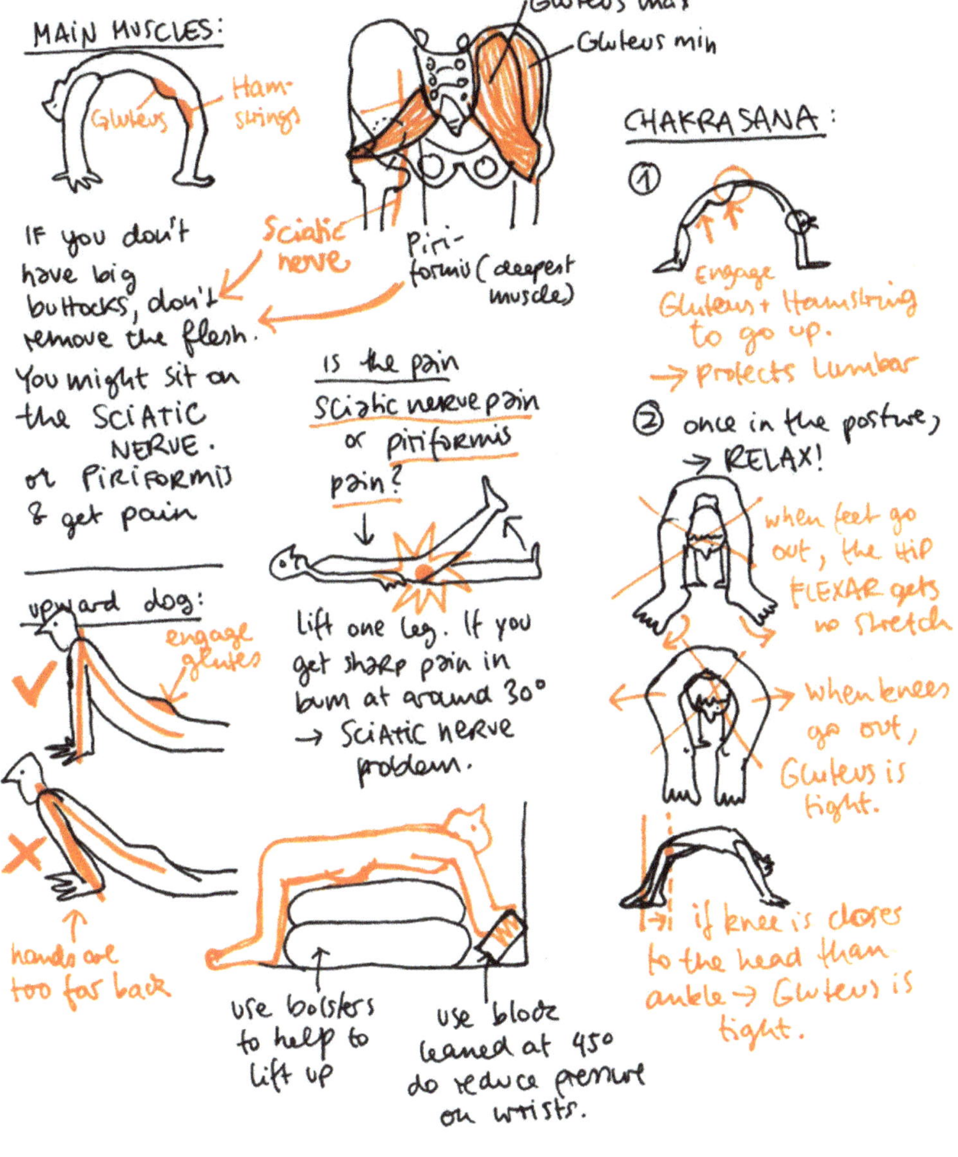

BACKWARD BENDING

MAIN MUSCLES:
Gluteus
Ham-strings

Gluteus max
Gluteus min

Sciatic nerve
Piri-formis (deepest muscle)

IF you don't have big buttocks, don't remove the flesh. You might sit on the SCIATIC NERVE. or PIRIFORMIS & get pain

upward dog:
engage glutes
✓
✗
hands are too far back

IS the pain
Sciatic nerve pain
or piriformis
pain?

Lift one leg. If you get sharp pain in bum at around 30° → Sciatic nerve problem.

use bolsters to help to lift up

use block leaned at 45° do reduce pressure on wrists.

CHAKRASANA:
① Engage Gluteus + Hamstring to go up.
→ Protects Lumbar
② once in the posture, → RELAX!

when feet go out, the HIP FLEXAR gets no stretch

When knees go out, Gluteus is tight.

if knee is closer to the head than ankle → Gluteus is tight.

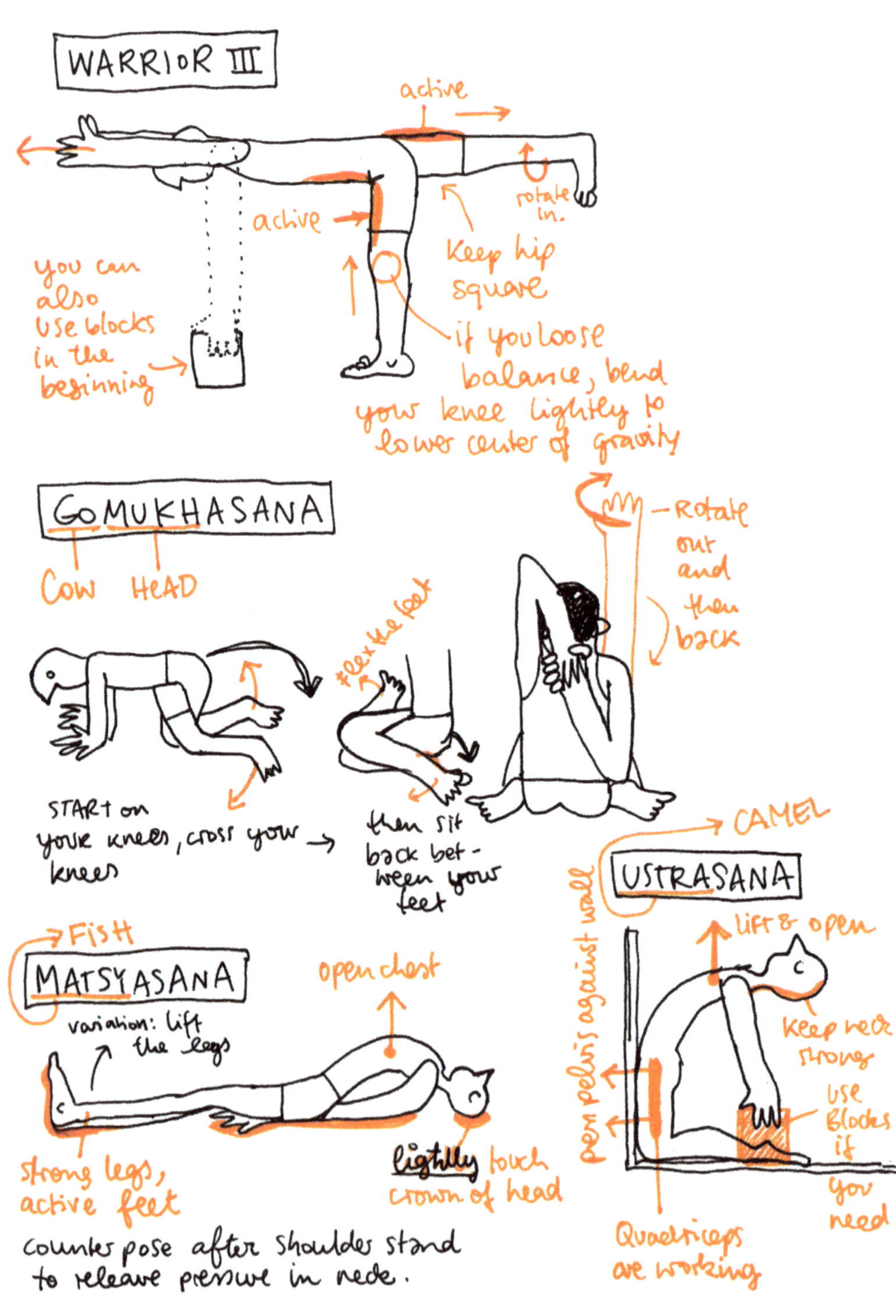

WARRIOR III
active
rotate in.
active
Keep hip square
if you loose balance, bend your knee lightly to lower center of gravity
you can also use blocks in the beginning
Rotate out and then back
GOMUKHASANA
COW HEAD
flex the feet
START on your knees, cross your knees
then sit back between your feet
CAMEL
USTRASANA
lift & open
press pelvis against wall
keep neck strong
use blocks if you need
Quadriceps are working
FISH
MATSYASANA
variation: lift the legs
open chest
lightly touch crown of head
strong legs, active feet
counter pose after shoulder stand to release pressure in neck.

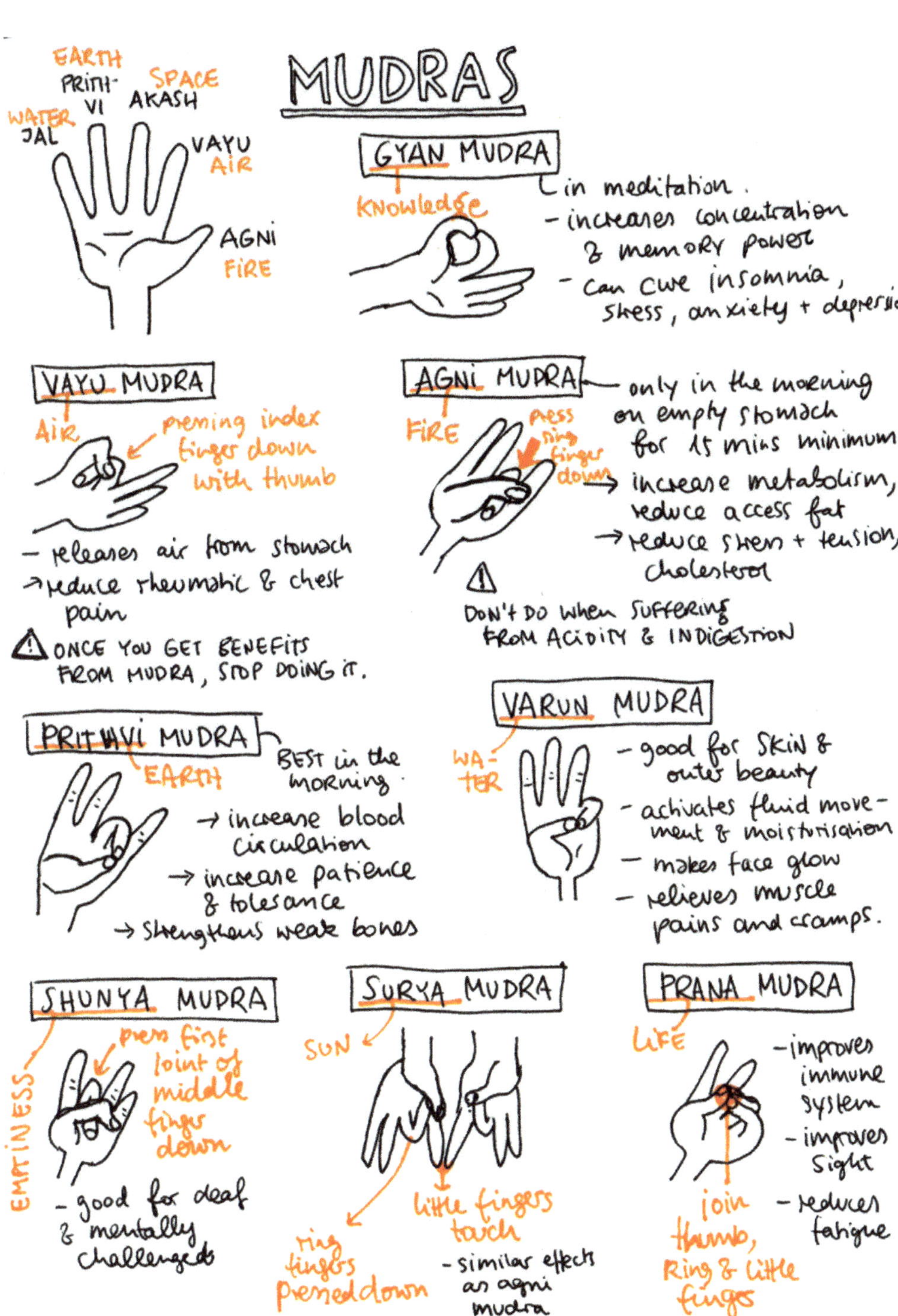

MUDRAS

EARTH
PRITH-VI
SPACE
AKASH
WATER
JAL
VAYU
AIR
AGNI
FIRE

GYAN MUDRA
KNOWLEDGE
- in meditation
- increases concentration & memory power
- can cure insomnia, stress, anxiety + depression

VAYU MUDRA
AIR
pressing index finger down with thumb
- releases air from stomach
- reduce rheumatic & chest pain
ONCE YOU GET BENEFITS FROM MUDRA, STOP DOING IT.

AGNI MUDRA
FIRE
press ring finger down
- only in the morning on empty stomach for 15 mins minimum
- increase metabolism, reduce access fat
- reduce stress + tension, cholesterol
DON'T DO WHEN SUFFERING FROM ACIDITY & INDIGESTION

PRITHVI MUDRA
EARTH
BEST in the morning
- increase blood circulation
- increase patience & tolerance
- strengthens weak bones

VARUN MUDRA
WATER
- good for SKIN & outer beauty
- activates fluid movement & moisturisation
- makes face glow
- relieves muscle pains and cramps.

SHUNYA MUDRA
EMPTINESS
press first joint of middle finger down
- good for deaf & mentally challenged

SURYA MUDRA
SUN
little fingers touch
ring finger pressed down
- similar effects as agni mudra

PRANA MUDRA
LIFE
- improves immune system
- improves sight
- reduces fatigue
join thumb, ring & little fingers

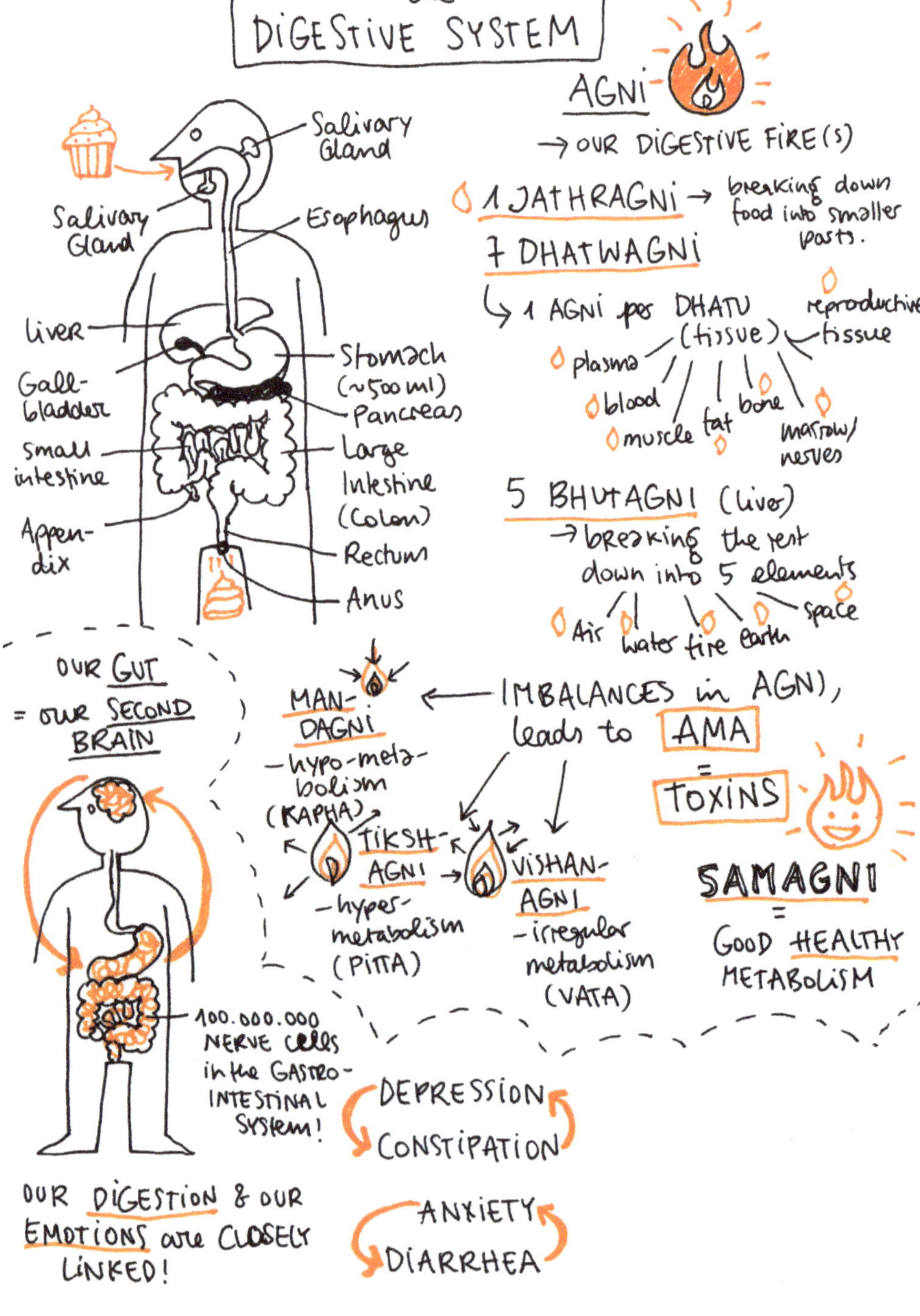

the DIGESTIVE SYSTEM

Salivary Gland
Salivary Gland
Esophagus
liver
Gall-bladder
small intestine
Appendix
Stomach (~500 ml)
Pancreas
Large Intestine (Colon)
Rectum
Anus

AGNI
→ OUR DIGESTIVE FIRE(S)

1 JATHRAGNI → breaking down food into smaller parts.

7 DHATWAGNI
↳ 1 AGNI per DHATU (tissue)
plasma
blood
muscle fat bone
reproductive tissue
marrow/ nerves

5 BHUTAGNI (liver)
→ breaking the rest down into 5 elements
Air water fire earth space

OUR GUT = OUR SECOND BRAIN

IMBALANCES in AGNI, leads to AMA = TOXINS

MAN-DAGNI
-hypo-meta-bolism (KAPHA)

TIKSH-AGNI
-hyper-metabolism (PITTA)

VISHAN-AGNI
-irregular metabolism (VATA)

SAMAGNI = GOOD HEALTHY METABOLISM

100.000.000 NERVE CELLS in the GASTRO-INTESTINAL System!

OUR DIGESTION & OUR EMOTIONS are CLOSELY LINKED!

DEPRESSION
CONSTIPATION
ANXIETY
DIARRHEA

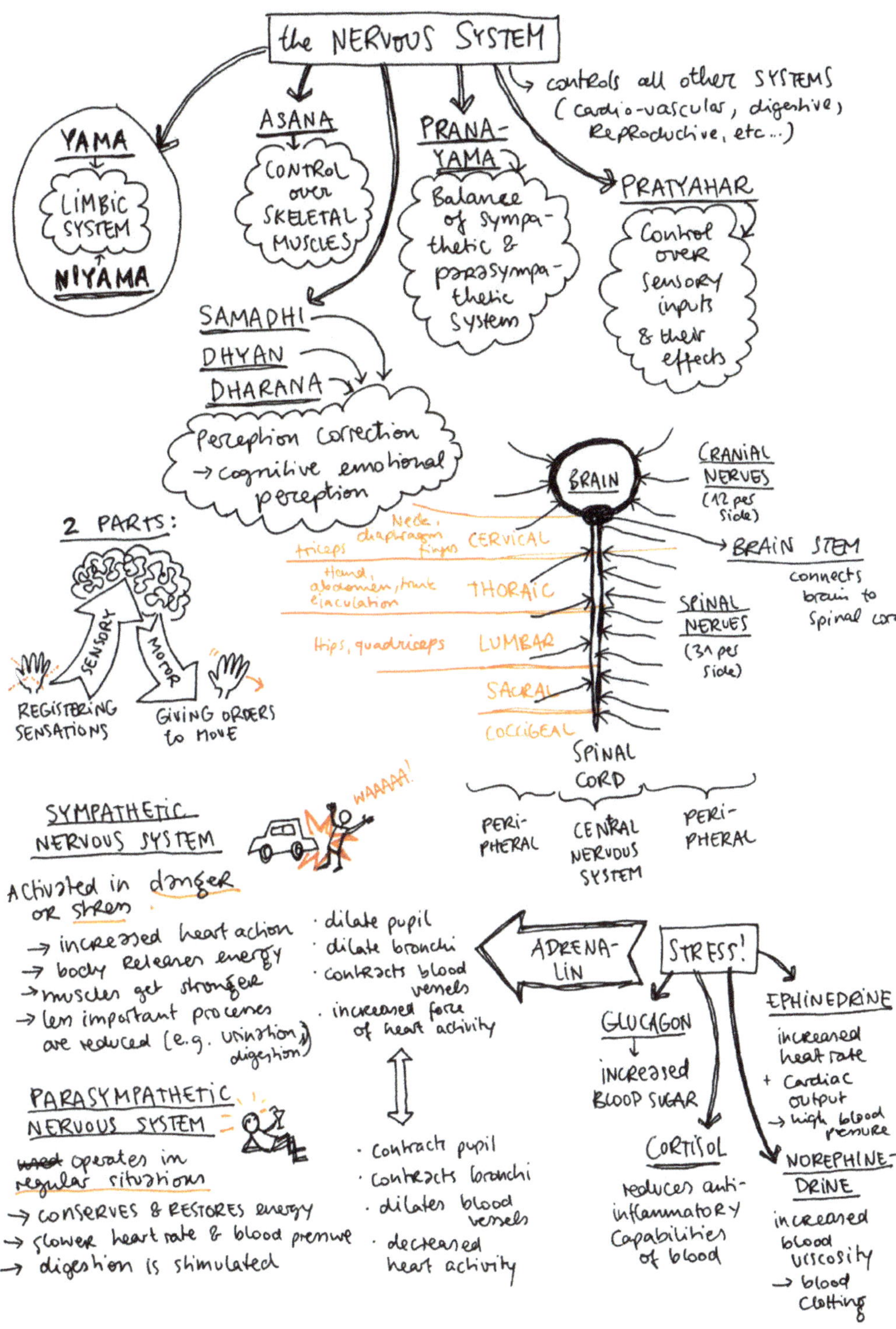
the NERVOUS SYSTEM

controls all other SYSTEMS
(cardio-vascular, digestive,
Reproductive, etc...)

YAMA
LIMBIC SYSTEM
NIYAMA

ASANA
CONTROL OVER SKELETAL MUSCLES

PRANA-YAMA
Balance of sympa-thetic & parasympa-thetic System

PRATYAHAR
Control over sensory inputs & their effects

SAMADHI
DHYAN
DHARANA

Perception correction
→ cognitive emotional perception

2 PARTS:

SENSORY
MOTOR

REGISTERING SENSATIONS

GIVING ORDERS to MOVE

BRAIN

CRANIAL NERVES
(12 per side)

Neck, diaphragm, fingers
triceps   CERVICAL

Hand, abdomen, trunk ejaculation   THORAIC

Hips, quadriceps   LUMBAR

SACRAL

COCCIGEAL

BRAIN STEM
connects brain to Spinal cord

SPINAL NERUES
(31 per side)

SPINAL CORD

PERI-PHERAL   CENTRAL NERVOUS SYSTEM   PERI-PHERAL

SYMPATHETIC NERVOUS SYSTEM

WAAAAAA!

Activated in danger or stress

→ increased heart action
→ body Releases energy
→ muscles get stronger
→ less important processes are reduced (e.g. urination, digestion)

· dilate pupil
· dilate bronchi
· contracts blood vessels
· increased force of heart activity

ADRENA-LIN   STRESS!

GLUCAGON
→ increased BLOOD SUGAR

CORTISOL
reduces anti-inflammatory capabilities of blood

EPHINEDRINE
increased heart rate + cardiac output → high blood pressure

NOREPHINE-DRINE
increased blood viscosity → blood clotting

PARASYMPATHETIC NERVOUS SYSTEM

operates in regular situations

→ CONSERVES & RESTORES energy
→ slower heart rate & blood pressure
→ digestion is stimulated

· contract pupil
· contracts bronchi
· dilates blood vessels
· decreased heart activity

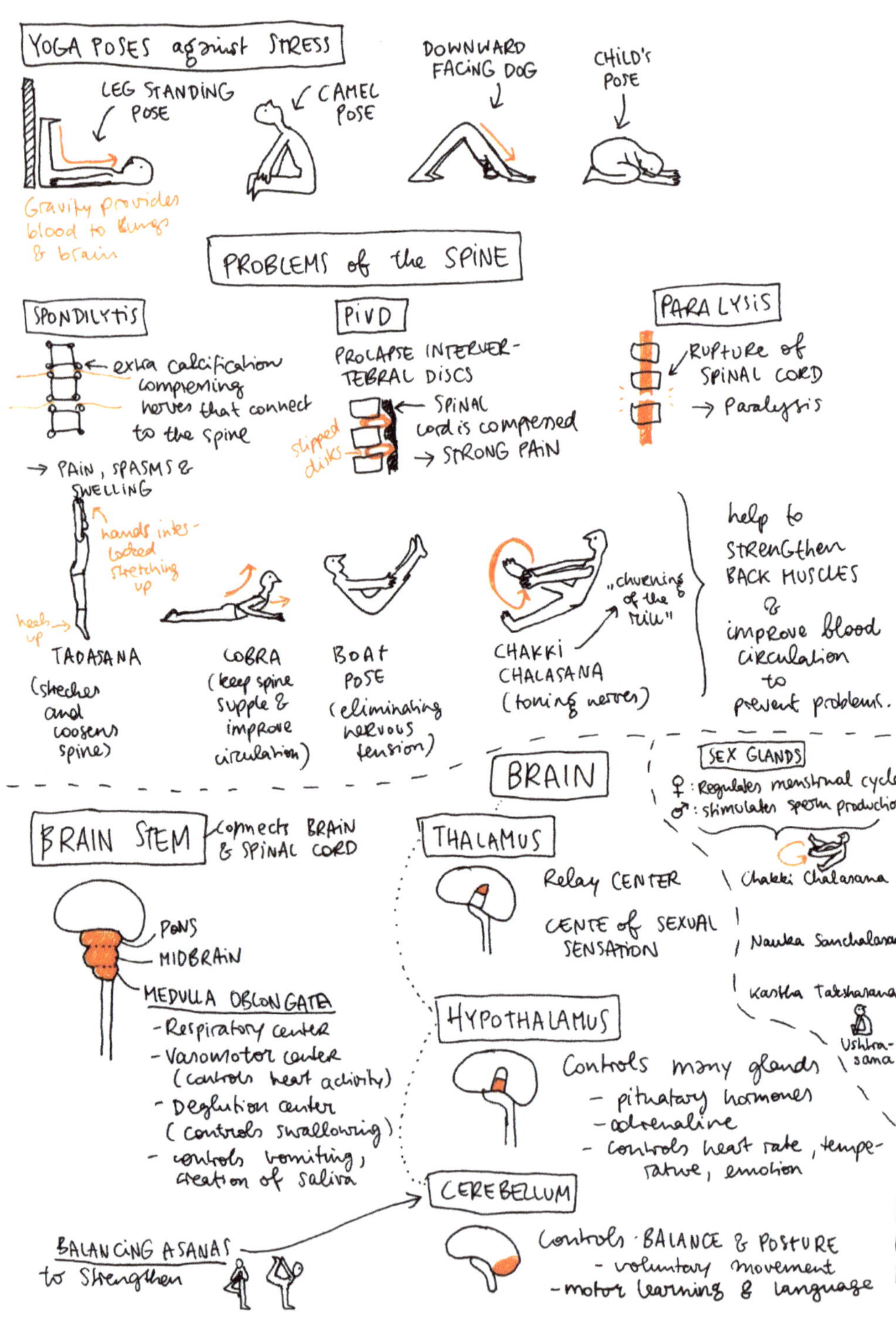

YOGA POSES against STRESS

LEG STANDING POSE
CAMEL POSE
DOWNWARD FACING DOG
CHILD'S POSE

Gravity provides blood to lungs & brain

PROBLEMS of the SPINE

SPONDILYTIS
extra calcification compressing nerves that connect to the spine
→ PAIN, SPASMS & SWELLING

hands inter-locked stretching up
heels up
TADASANA
(streches and loosens spine)

COBRA
(keep spine supple & improve circulation)

BOAT POSE
(eliminating nervous tension)

PIVD
PROLAPSE INTERVERTEBRAL DISCS
slipped disks
SPINAL cord is compressed
→ STRONG PAIN

CHAKKI CHALASANA
(toning nerves)
"churning of the mill"

PARALYSIS
RUPTURE of SPINAL CORD
→ Paralysis

help to STRENGTHEN BACK MUSCLES & improve blood circulation to prevent problems.

BRAIN

SEX GLANDS
♀: Regulates menstrual cycle
♂: stimulates sperm production
Chakki Chalasana
Nauka Sanchalasana
Kastha Takshasana
Ushtrasana

BRAIN STEM
connect BRAIN & SPINAL CORD
PONS
MIDBRAIN
MEDULLA OBLONGATE
- Respiratory center
- Vasomotor center (controls heart activity)
- Deglution center (controls swallowing)
- controls vomiting, creation of saliva

BALANCING ASANAS to Strengthen

THALAMUS
Relay CENTER
CENTE of SEXUAL SENSATION

HYPOTHALAMUS
Controls many glands
- pituatary hormones
- adrenaline
- controls heart rate, temperature, emotion

CEREBELLUM
Controls BALANCE & POSTURE
- voluntary movement
- motor learning & language

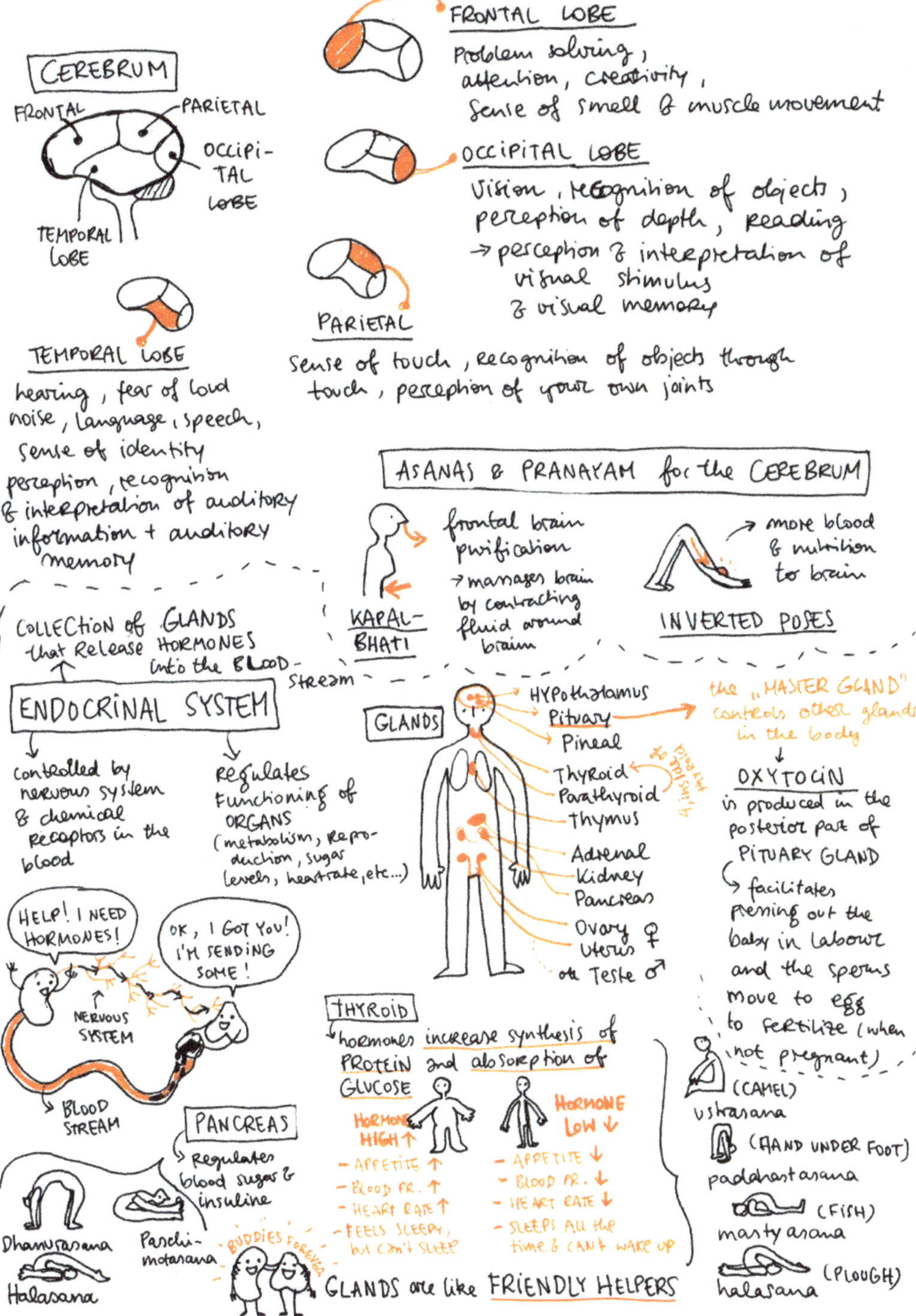

CEREBRUM
FRONTAL
PARIETAL
OCCIPITAL LOBE
TEMPORAL LOBE

FRONTAL LOBE
Problem solving, attention, creativity, sense of smell & muscle movement

OCCIPITAL LOBE
Vision, recognition of objects, perception of depth, reading
→ perception & interpretation of visual stimulus & visual memory

PARIETAL
Sense of touch, recognition of objects through touch, perception of your own joints

TEMPORAL LOBE
hearing, fear of loud noise, language, speech, sense of identity perception, recognition & interpretation of auditory information + auditory memory

ASANAS & PRANAYAM for the CEREBRUM
KAPAL-BHATI
frontal brain purification
→ massages brain by contracting fluid around brain
INVERTED POSES
→ more blood & nutrition to brain

COLLECTION OF GLANDS that Release HORMONES into the BLOOD-stream

ENDOCRINAL SYSTEM
controlled by nervous system & chemical receptors in the blood
regulates functioning of ORGANS (metabolism, reproduction, sugar levels, heartrate, etc...)

HELP! I NEED HORMONES!
OK, I GOT YOU! I'M SENDING SOME!
NERVOUS SYSTEM
BLOOD STREAM

GLANDS
HYPOTHALAMUS
Pituary
Pineal
Thyroid
Parathyroid
Thymus
Adrenal
Kidney
Pancreas
Ovary ♀
Uterus ♀
or Teste ♂
please protect

the „MASTER GLAND" controls other glands in the body
OXYTOCIN
is produced in the posterior part of PITUARY GLAND
↳ facilitates pushing out the baby in labour and the sperm move to egg to fertilize (when not pregnant)

(CAMEL) ustrasana
(HAND UNDER FOOT) padahastasana
(FISH) matsyasana
(PLOUGH) halasana

THYROID
hormones increase synthesis of PROTEIN and absorption of GLUCOSE
HORMONE HIGH ↑
- APPETITE ↑
- BLOOD PR. ↑
- HEART RATE ↑
- FEELS SLEEPY, but can't sleep
HORMONE LOW ↓
- APPETITE ↓
- BLOOD PR. ↓
- HEART RATE ↓
- SLEEPS ALL THE time & CAN'T WAKE UP

PANCREAS
→ regulates blood sugar & insuline
Dhanurasana
Paschimotanasana
Halasana
BUDDIES FOREVER
GLANDS are like FRIENDLY HELPERS

AYURVEDA

→ PHYSICAL, MENTAL & SOCIAL

LIFE · KNOWLEDGE

KNOWLEDGE of LIFE
→ first you need to KNOW YOURSELF

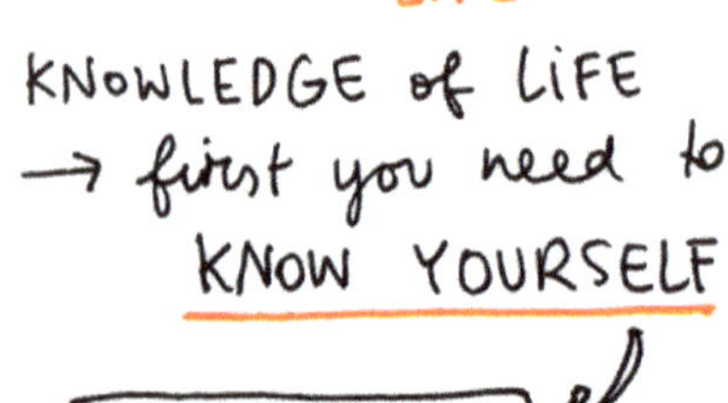

TRIDOSHA

3 · ENERGY

↳ 3 subtle energies which can be disturbed

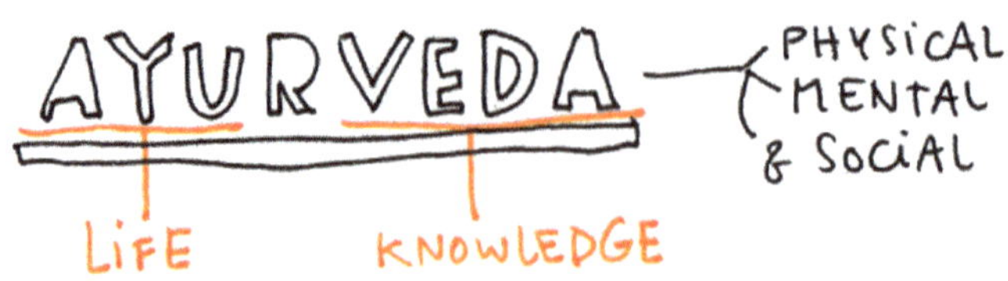

PANCH MAHA BHUTA —

5 · BIG · ELEMENTS

- 🪨 PRITHUI – EARTH
- 💧 JAL – WATER
- 🔥 AGNI – FIRE
- 🌬 VAYU – AIR
- ✦ AKASH – SPACE

all living & non-living things are made out of these five.

VATA = AIR + SPACE

→ **movement**
(when we are dead, VATA is gone)

→ DRY, LIGHT, COLD, MOBILE, ERRATIC, SUBTLE, ASTRIGENT

slim, loosing weight is easy, gain weight on belly & face

cold hands & feet, poor blood circulation

irregular habits, should eat + sleep regularly, get bored easily

avoid conflicts, feel anxiety, stress & worries

dry skin, hair + colon → constipation

very active, many kinds of thoughts in mind

taste of vata → drying & choking taste (e.g. all unripe fruit, turmeric, cloves)

Good tastes for VATA:
SWEET, SOUR, SALT

Not good:
ASTRIGENT, PUNGENT, BITTER

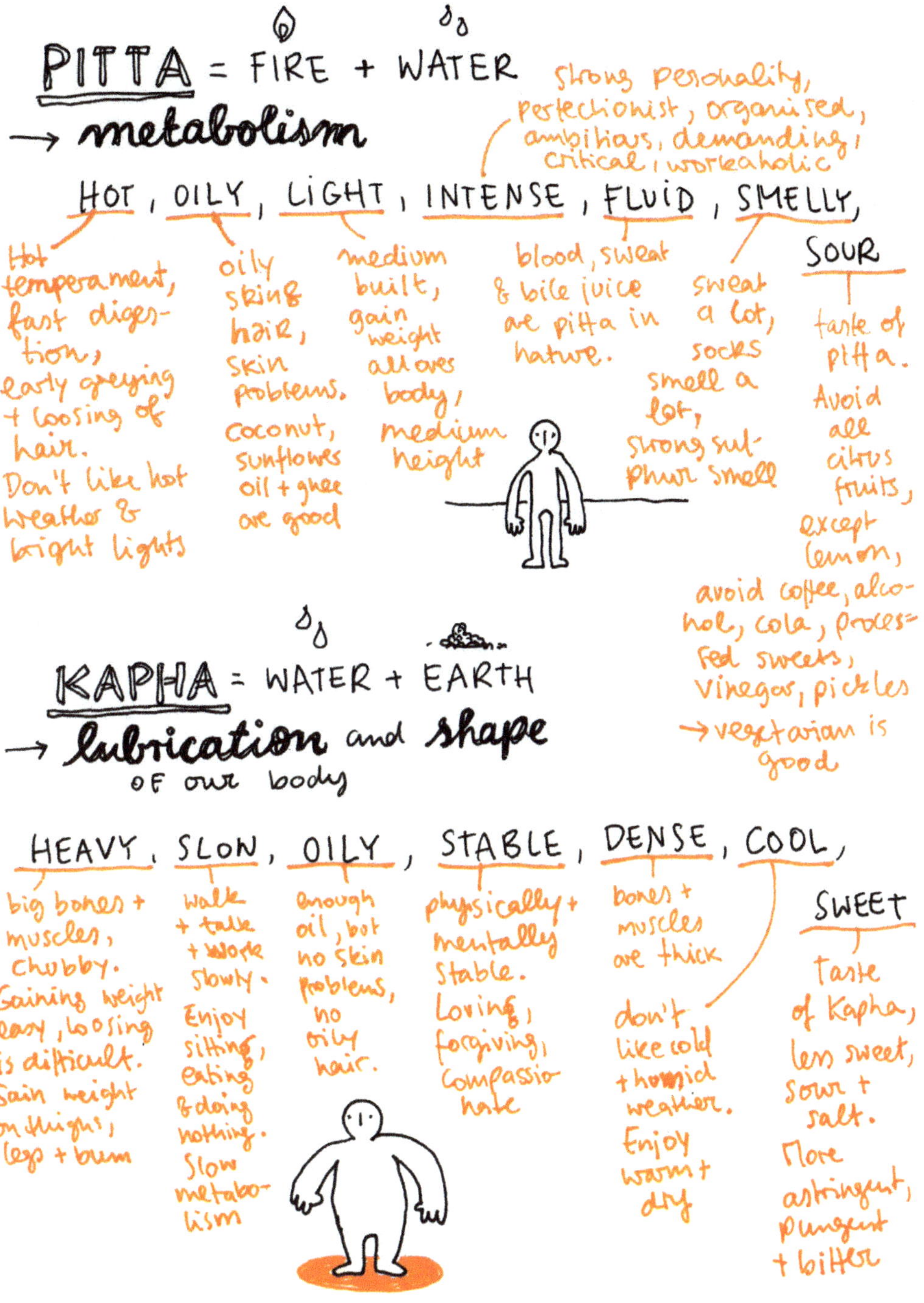# PITTA = FIRE + WATER

→ *metabolism*

strong personality, perfectionist, organised, ambitious, demanding, critical, workaholic

HOT, OILY, LIGHT, INTENSE, FLUID, SMELLY, SOUR

Hot
Hot temperament, fast digestion, early greying + loosing of hair.
Don't like hot weather & bright lights

Oily
oily skin& hair, skin problems.
Coconut, sunflower oil + ghee are good

Light
medium built, gain weight all over body, medium height

Intense
blood, sweat & bile juice are pitta in nature.

Fluid
sweat a lot, socks smell a lot, strong sulphur smell

Sour
taste of pitta. Avoid all citrus fruits, except lemon, avoid coffee, alcohol, cola, processed sweets, vinegar, pickles
→ vegetarian is good

KAPHA = WATER + EARTH

→ *lubrication* and *shape* of our body

HEAVY, SLOW, OILY, STABLE, DENSE, COOL, SWEET

Heavy
big bones + muscles, chubby. Gaining weight easy, loosing is difficult. Gain weight on thighs, legs + bum

Slow
walk + talk + work slowly. Enjoy sitting, eating & doing nothing. Slow metabolism

Oily
enough oil, but no skin problems, no oily hair.

Stable
physically + mentally stable. Loving, forgiving, compassionate

Dense
bones + muscles are thick
don't like cold + humid weather. Enjoy warm + dry

Sweet
taste of Kapha, less sweet, sour + salt. More astringent, pungent + bitter

PRAKRITI → YOUR INDIVIDUAL CONSTITUTION

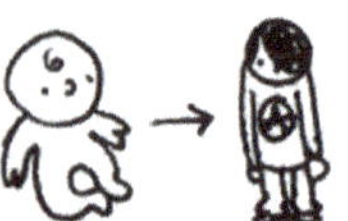

FROM BIRTH to PUBERTY: **KAPHA** is HIGH
(immune + respiratory system)

decided at the time of conception

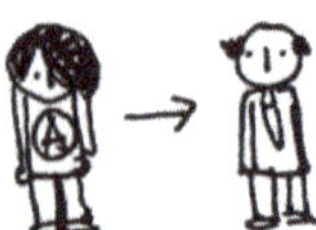

FROM PUBERTY to ~50 YEARS OLD: **PITTA** is HIGH
(digestive system, skin, blood, urinal, genital, endocrine system, heart, liver, spleen)

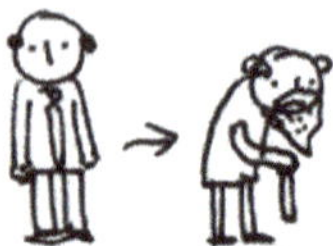

50 YEARS ONWARDS: **VATA** is HIGH
(musculo-skeletal, nervous system, mental problems)

7 TYPES of PRAKRITI

ONE DOSHA

① VATA (>60%)

② PITTA (>60%)

③ KAPHA (>60%)

very rare types

TWO DOSHA

most common

④ VATA-PITTA ●●●

⑤ VATA-KAPHA ●●

⑥ PITTA-KAPHA ●

very common types

THREE DOSHA

⑦ SAM or TRIDOSHAJ
= same level
(each dosha ~30-40%)

very rare type

VIKRITI → the DISTURBANCES

↳ PULSE DIAGNOSIS ①

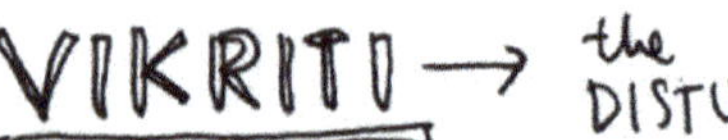

↓ on both hands & on empty stomach
(~3 hours no food)

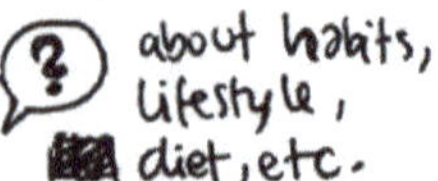

VIKRITI ANALYSIS
→ find out the IMBALANCES

② OBSERVATION

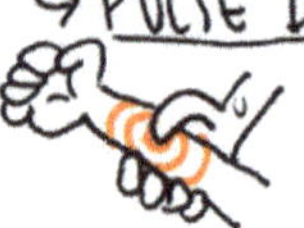

← Body constitution, hair, teeth, skin, etc...

③ QUESTIONS

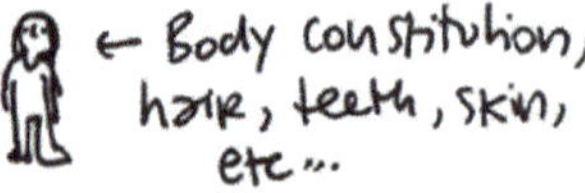

PRAKRITI ANALYSIS

① BUILD:
Vata – Tall or short & slim
Pitta – Medium
Kapha – Chubby, tall & big

② SKIN:
V: Darker than other family members, dry
P: more pink & oily
K: more white & normal

③ HAIR:
V: thin, dry, brittle, lot, brown
P: thin, oily, straight, less, early greying + loosing, light
K: thick, curly, a lot, not dry nor oily, dark colour

④ WEIGHT GAINING:
V: gaining hard, loosing easy
P: gaining & loosing easy
K: gaining easy, loosing difficult

⑤ WEIGHT GAINING PART:
V: Belly + face
P: everywhere
K: Thighs + bum

⑥ TALKING:
V: a lot + fast
P: medium, selective
K: less + slowly

⑦ WALKING:
V: fast
P: medium
K: slow

⑧ EYES:
V: small
P: medium
K: big

⑨ SLEEP:
V: 7-8 hours, light, morning: takes time to get up
P: 5-6 hours, deep, get up immediately
K: enjoy sleeping

⑩ DREAMS:
V: Nightmares, stressful dreams, running, flying
P: strong, spiritual, realistic, conflicts, adventurous, fire
K: routine, water

⑪ CHILDHOOD:
V: slim, small, shy, mostly healthy
P: medium, open, mostly healthy
K: chubby, silent, can have respiratory problems frequently

⑫ TEMPERAMENT:
V: easily get stressed
P: strong
K: relaxed

⑬ CONFLICTS:
V: avoid, run away
P: resolve ASAP
K: loving, forgiving

⑭ DISEASES:
V: constipation, dry skin, joint pains, hypertension
P: skin problem, hepatitis, heart problems, cancer, urine/genital infections, acidity
K: diabetes, obesity, respiratory, immune problems

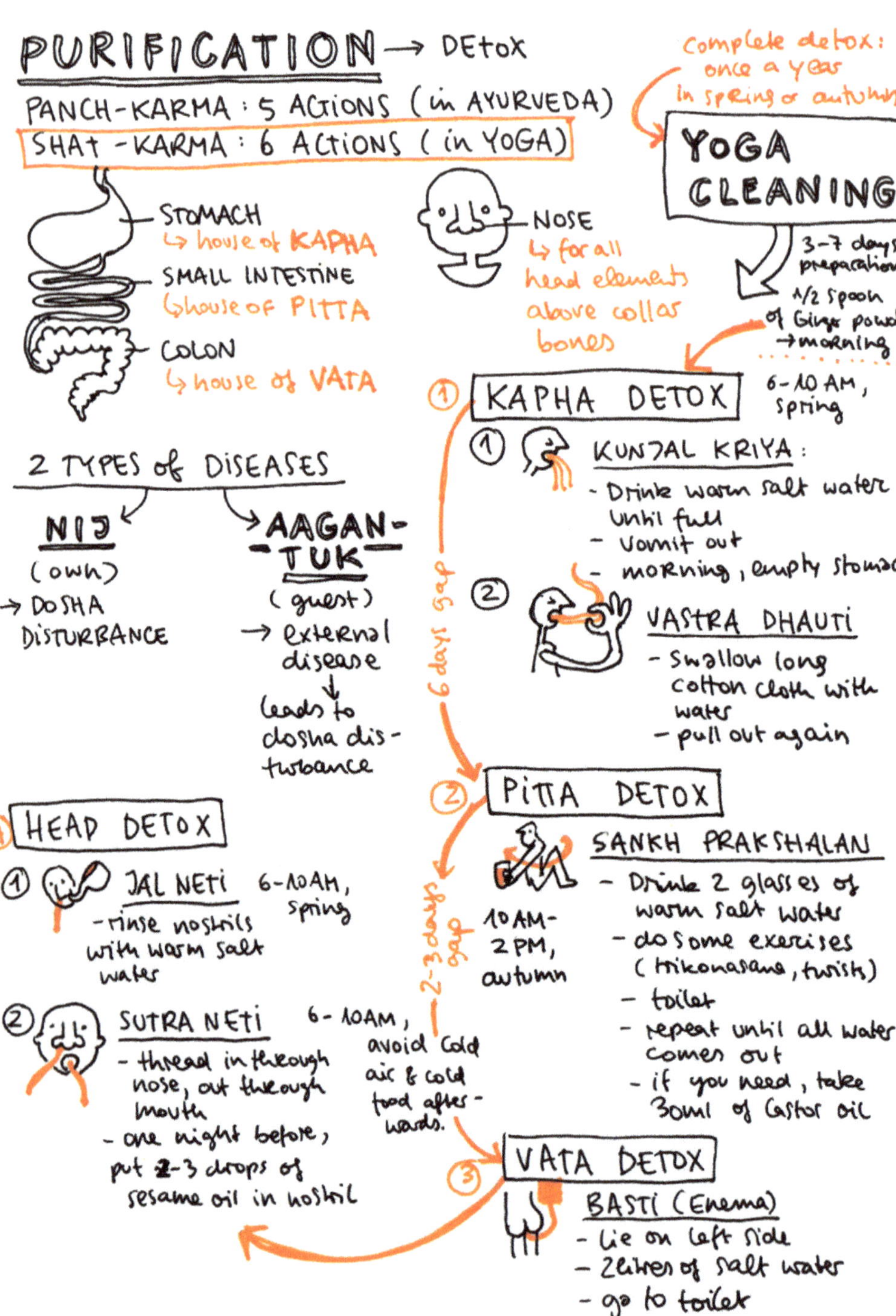

PURIFICATION → DETOX
PANCH-KARMA : 5 ACTIONS (in AYURVEDA)
SHAt - KARMA : 6 ACTIONS (in YOGA)

STOMACH
↳ house of KAPHA
SMALL INTESTINE
↳ house of PITTA
COLON
↳ house of VATA

NOSE
↳ for all head elements above collar bones

complete detox: once a year in spring or autumn

YOGA CLEANING

3-7 days preparation:
1/2 spoon of Ginger powder → morning
6-10 AM, spring

2 TYPES of DISEASES
NIJ
(own)
→ DOSHA DISTURBANCE
AAGAN-TUK
(guest)
→ external disease
↓
leads to dosha dis-turbance

① KAPHA DETOX
① KUNJAL KRIYA :
- Drink warm salt water until full
- Vomit out
- morning, empty stomach
② VASTRA DHAUTI
- Swallow long cotton cloth with water
- pull out again

6 days gap

② PITTA DETOX
SANKH PRAKSHALAN
10AM-2PM, autumn
- Drink 2 glasses of warm salt water
- do some exercises (trikonasana, twists)
- toilet
- repeat until all water comes out
- if you need, take 30ml of castor oil

④ HEAD DETOX
① JAL NETI 6-10AM, spring
- rinse nostrils with warm salt water
② SUTRA NETI 6-10AM, avoid cold air & cold food after-wards.
- thread in through nose, out through mouth
- one night before, put 2-3 drops of sesame oil in nostril

2-3 days gap

③ VATA DETOX
BASTI (Enema)
- Lie on left side
- 2 liters of salt water
- go to toilet

YOGA PHILOSOPHY

TAUGHT BY
VIMAL SHARMA

PURUSHA

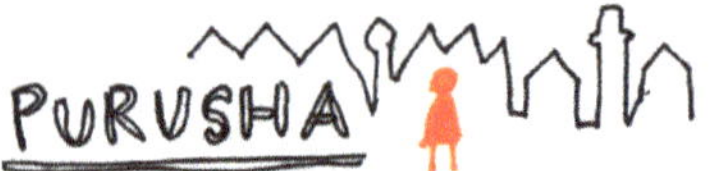

LITERALLY: „the DWELLER of the CITY" ↓

think of the body & mind as the cities

the **TRUE PERSON** within

the **SOUL** or **SPIRIT**

→ THE **SEER**, the WITNESS

→ SPIRITUAL <u>CONSCIOUS</u> FORCE

CONCIOUSNESS

... UNCHANGING & UNCAUSED (*like nature's laws*)

the MIND is a REFLECTION of PURUSHA

←(PURUSHA) SUN

↑ MIRROR (MIND) → VIKRTI

PRAKRTI

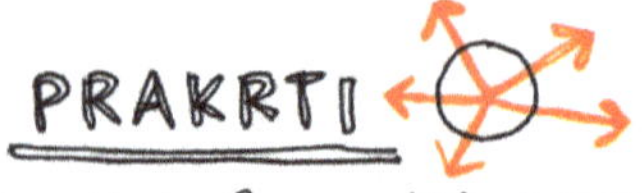

LITERALLY: „ that from which SOMETHING ORIGINATES " ↓

the **ORIGIN** of EVERYTHING, the ultimate **CAUSE** of this UNIVERSE

→ WHAT is **SEEN**

→ <u>unconscious</u> MATERIAL FORCE

PURPOSE

PRAKRTi has no purpose on its own, it needs to be witnessed by Purusha

MATTER

... the <u>unmanifest</u> form of matter, untangible

(**VIKRTI** → the <u>MANIFEST</u> form of matter ... all objects, things, our body, our <u>mind</u>)

SEED: <u>PRAKRTi</u>
(*Seed has the potential of the tree but is not manifested yet*)

TREE: <u>VIKRiTi</u>
The actual manifested tree once it is grown

SELF REALISATION:

SATTVA — when the lake is still + clear, I can see my reflection

RAJAS — when there are waves, I can't see my Re-flection

if the lake is muddy, I can't see my reflection — TAMAS

in meditation, we are trying to create more and more SATTVA. At the peak of SATTVA there is <u>self-realisation</u>

SEED: PRAKRTi
TREE: VIKRiTi

SATTVA
LIGHT

RAJAS
MOVEMENT

TAMAS
INERTIA

PRAKRiTi is when there 3 Forces are in perfect equilibrium

" MEDITATION is not about DOING... when the DOING ENDS, the meditation starts "

MEDITATION is **STATE**, not **PROCESS.**

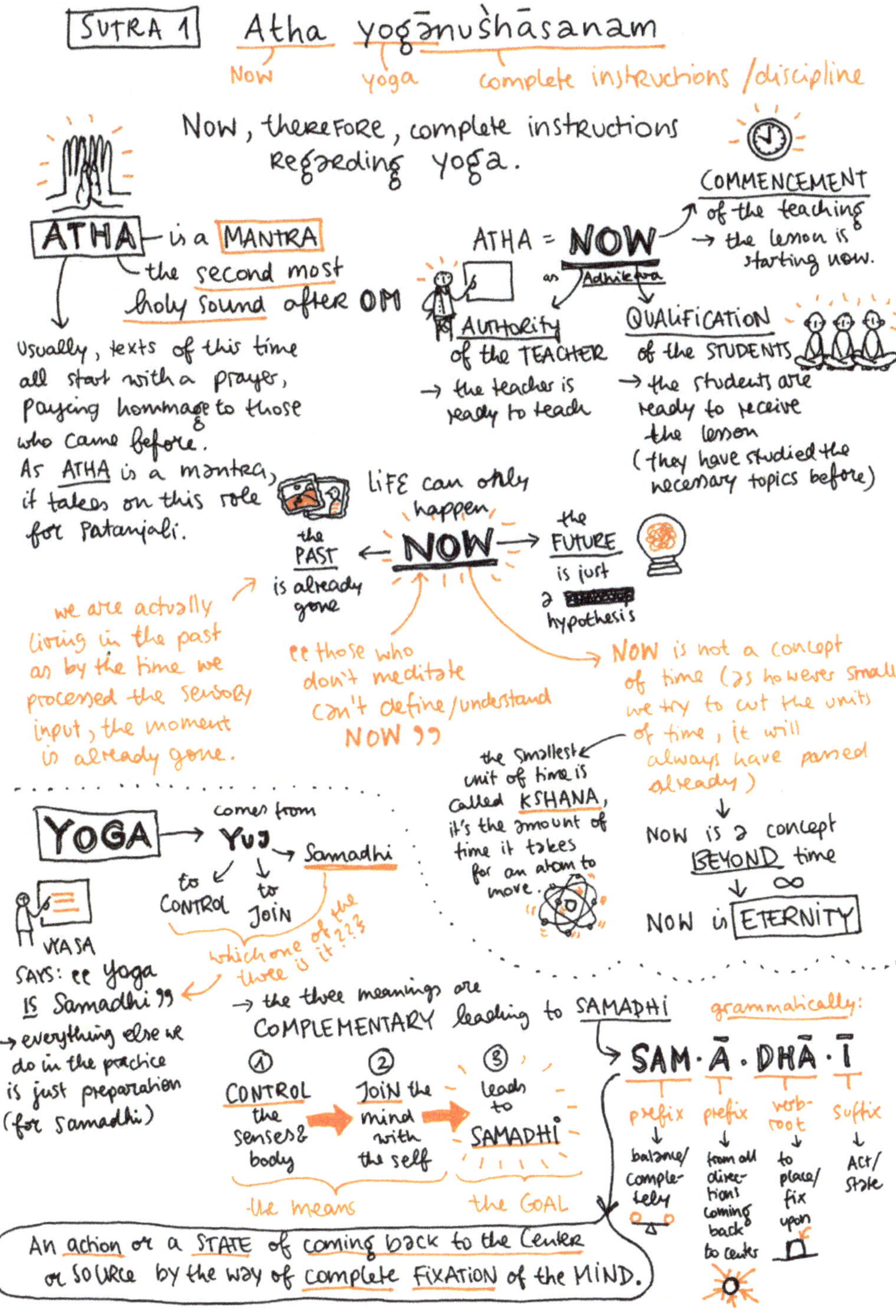

SUTRA 1   Atha yogānushāsanam
Now   yoga   complete instructions / discipline

Now, therefore, complete instructions regarding yoga.

ATHA is a MANTRA
the second most holy sound after OM

COMMENCEMENT
of the teaching
→ the lesson is starting now.

ATHA = NOW
an Adhikara

Usually, texts of this time all start with a prayer, paying hommage to those who came before.
As ATHA is a mantra, it takes on this role for Patanjali.

AUTHORITY of the TEACHER
→ the teacher is ready to teach

QUALIFICATION of the STUDENTS
→ the students are ready to receive the lesson
(they have studied the necessary topics before)

LIFE can only happen
the PAST ← NOW → the FUTURE
is already gone
is just a hypothesis

we are actually living in the past as by the time we processed the sensory input, the moment is already gone.

"those who don't meditate can't define/understand NOW"

NOW is not a concept of time (as however small we try to cut the units of time, it will always have passed already)
↓
NOW is a concept BEYOND time
↓ ∞
NOW is ETERNITY

the smallest unit of time is called KSHANA, it's the amount of time it takes for an atom to move.

YOGA → comes from → YUJ → Samadhi
to CONTROL
to JOIN
which one of the three is it???

VYASA SAYS: "yoga IS Samadhi"
→ everything else we do in the practice is just preparation (for samadhi)

→ the three meanings are COMPLEMENTARY leading to SAMADHI

grammatically:

① CONTROL the senses & body
② JOIN the mind with the self
③ leads to SAMADHI

the means   the GOAL

SAM · Ā · DHĀ · Ī
prefix   prefix   verb-root   suffix
↓   ↓   ↓   ↓
balance/ from all to place/   ACT/
comple-   direc-   fix   state
tely   tions   upon
          coming
          back
          to centre

An action or a STATE of coming back to the center or SOURCE by the way of complete FIXATION of the MIND.

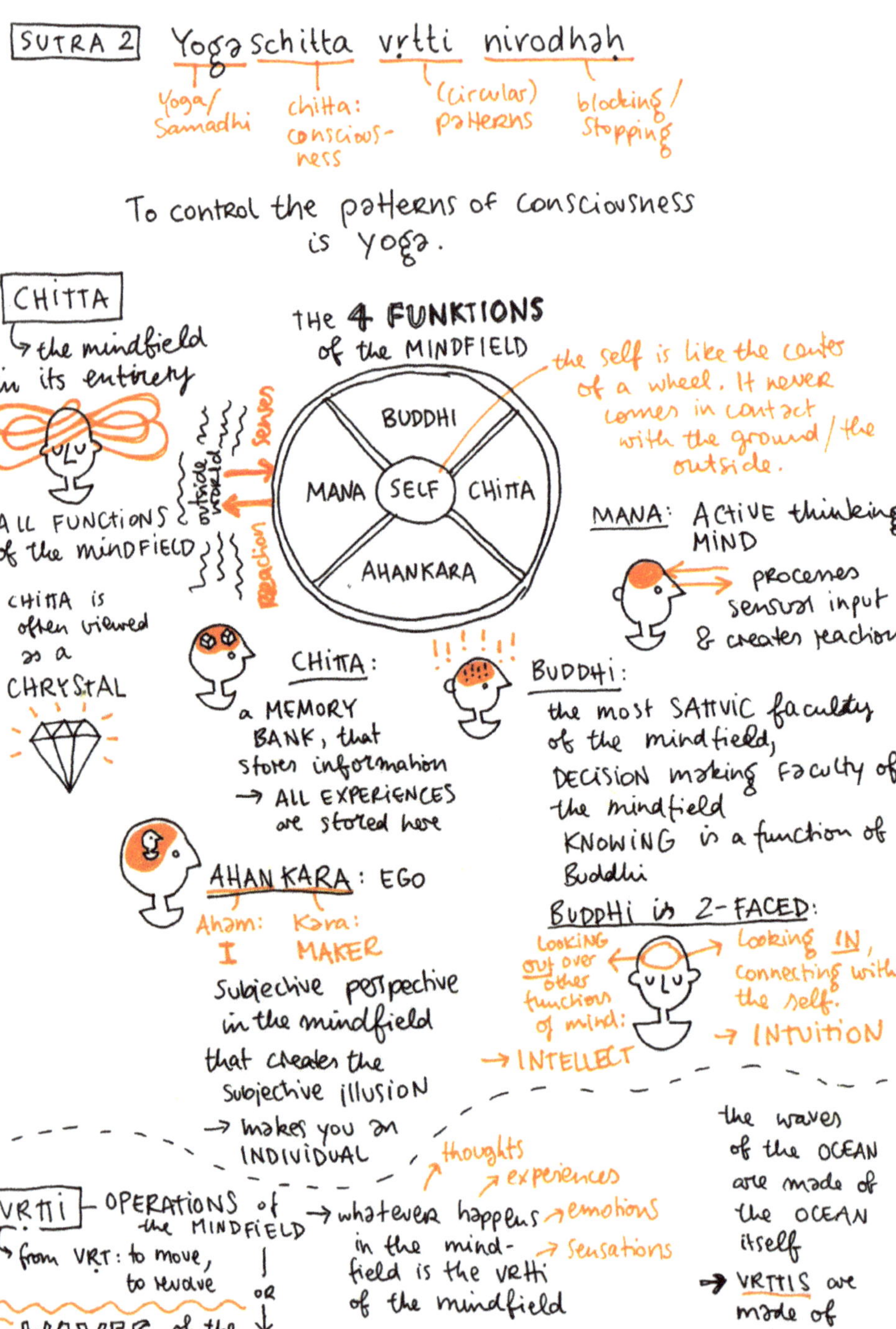

SUTRA 2 | Yogaschitta vṛtti nirodhaḥ

Yoga/ Samadhi
chitta: consciousness
(circular) patterns
blocking/ stopping

To control the patterns of consciousness is yoga.

CHITTA
↳ the mindfield in its entirety

ALL FUNCTIONS of the MINDFIELD

CHITTA is often viewed as a CHRYSTAL

THE 4 FUNKTIONS of the MINDFIELD

outside world
senses
reaction

BUDDHI
MANA   SELF   CHITTA
AHANKARA

the self is like the center of a wheel. It never comes in contact with the ground/ the outside.

MANA: ACTIVE thinking MIND
→ processes sensual input & creates reaction

CHITTA:
a MEMORY BANK, that stores information
→ ALL EXPERIENCES are stored here

BUDDHI:
the most SATTVIC faculty of the mindfield,
DECISION making faculty of the mindfield
KNOWING is a function of Buddhi

AHANKARA: EGO

Aham: Kara:
I   MAKER

subjective perspective in the mindfield
that creates the subjective illusion
→ makes you an INDIVIDUAL

BUDDHI is 2-FACED:
looking out over other functions of mind:
→ INTELLECT
Looking IN, connecting with the self.
→ INTUITION

thoughts
→ experiences

the waves of the OCEAN are made of the OCEAN itself

VRTTI — OPERATIONS of the MINDFIELD
↳ from VRT: to move, to revolve
or
WAVES of the mindfield

→ whatever happens in the mind-field is the vṛtti of the mindfield
→ emotions
→ sensations

→ VRTTIS are made of CHITTA

NIRODHA → the full CONTROL of the MINDFIELD ≠ SUPPRESSION or BLOCKING

NI · RUDH

UNDER — to restrain / to control

Control means UNDERSTANDING ⟷ SUPPRESSION needs too much force & it only works temporarily

so you can master it without force

(which is SAMADHI)

⇒ YOGA is the CONTROL of the MODIFI-CATIONS of the MINDFIELD

π YOGA is the DESOLUTION of the VRTTIS back into the MINDFIELD.

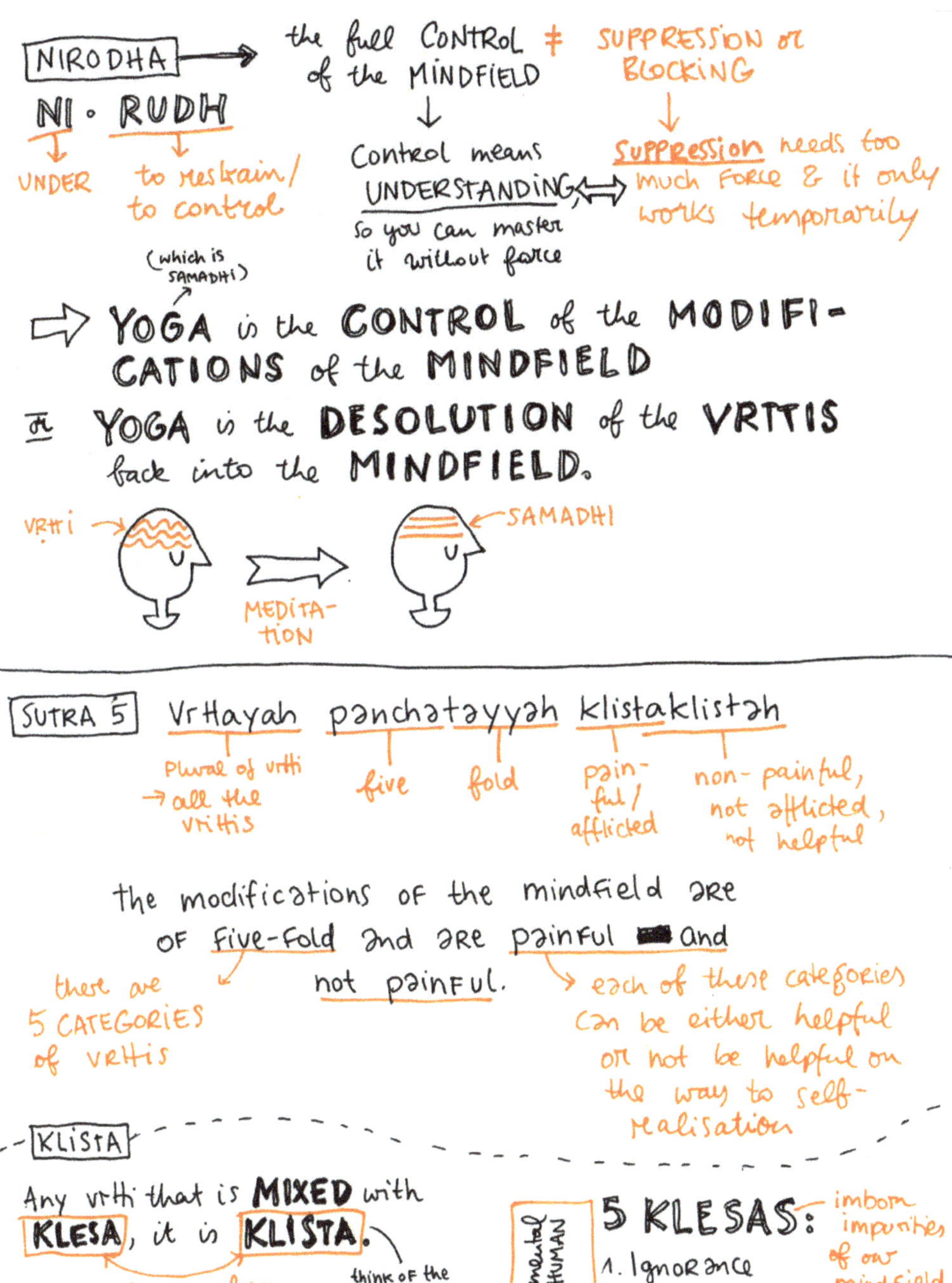

SUTRA 5 — Vrttayah panchatayyah klistaklistah

Plural of vritti → all the vrittis

five

fold

painful / afflicted

non-painful, not afflicted, not helpful

the modifications of the mindfield are of five-fold and are painful and not painful.

there are 5 CATEGORIES of vrittis

→ each of these categories can be either helpful or not be helpful on the way to self-realisation

KLISTA

Any vrtti that is MIXED with KLESA, it is KLISTA.

words come from the same root.

think of the opposite

All other vrttis are AKLISTA → pure KNOWLEDGE / full REALISATION

the 5 fundamental Reason for HUMAN SUFFERING

5 KLESAS: — inborn impurities of our mindfield
1. Ignorance
2. Ego
3. Attachment
4. Hatred / Aversion
5. Fear

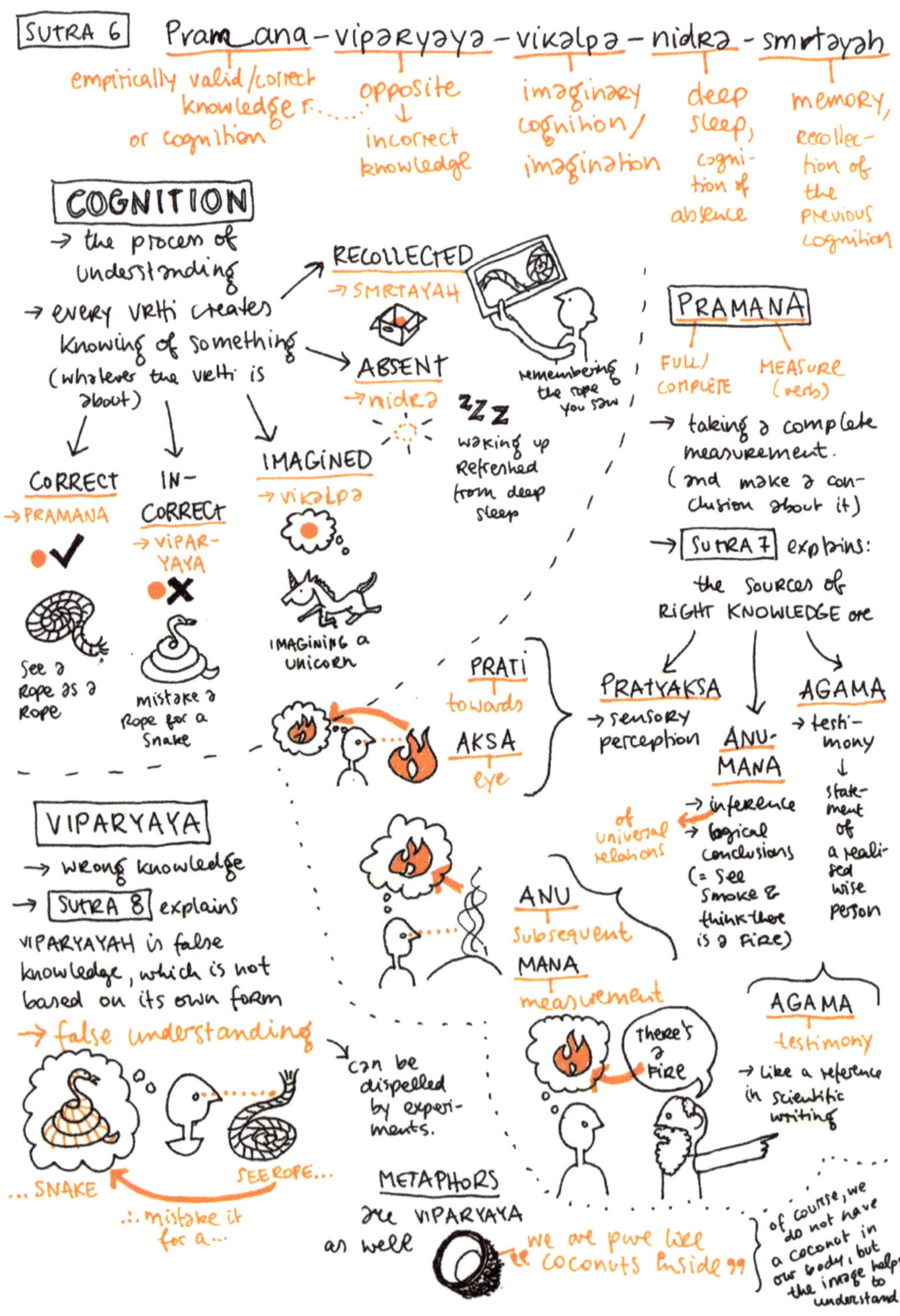

SUTRA 6 Pram_ana - viparyaya - vikalpa - nidra - smrtayah

empirically valid/correct knowledge r. or cognition
opposite → incorrect knowledge
imaginary cognition / imagination
deep sleep, cognition of absence
memory, recollection of the previous cognition

COGNITION
→ the process of understanding
→ every vrtti creates knowing of something (whatever the vrtti is about)

RECOLLECTED
→ SMRTAYAH
ABSENT
→ nidra
remembering the rope you saw
ZZZ
waking up refreshed from deep sleep

CORRECT
→ PRAMANA
✔
See a Rope as a Rope

IN-CORRECT
→ VIPAR-YAYA
✘
mistake a Rope for a Snake

IMAGINED
→ vikalpa
IMAGINING a Unicorn

PRAMANA
FULL/COMPLETE
MEASURE (verb)
→ taking a complete measurement. (and make a con- clusion about it)
→ SUTRA 7 explains: the sources of RIGHT KNOWLEDGE are

PRATI towards
AKSA eye

PRATYAKSA
→ sensory perception

ANU- MANA
→ inference
→ logical conclusions (= see smoke & think there is a fire)
of universal relations

AGAMA
→ testi- mony
↓
state- ment of a reali- sed wise person

VIPARYAYA
→ wrong knowledge
→ SUTRA 8 explains
VIPARYAYAH is false knowledge, which is not based on its own form
→ false understanding

... SNAKE
... mistake it for a...
SEE ROPE...

can be dispelled by experi- ments.

ANU subsequent
MANA measurement
there's a fire

AGAMA testimony
→ like a reference in scientific writing

METAPHORS are VIPARYAYA as well
we are pure like coconuts inside

of course, we do not have a coconut in our body, but the image helps to understand.

VIKALPA
→ IMAGINATION
→ **SUTRA 9** explains:
dependent upon a
verbal knowledge only,
but devoid of any such
object is imagination
→ NOT CREATIVE
IMAGINATION, but
just having nothing to do
with reality

NIDRA → subconscious
state of mind
→ DEEP SLEEP
→ **SUTRA 10** explains:
SLEEP is the modification
of the mindfield based
on the COGNITION of
ABSENCE.

ABSENCE does not
exist. It is a
paradox CONCEPT.

SMRITI
→ MEMORY
SUTRA 11 explains:
Not letting the experienced
objects escape from the
mind is MEMORY.
↓
EXPERIENCE
gives rise to
MEMORY

all language is VIKALPA in
some way, because a word is
≠ APPLE not the OBJECT but
an arbitrary
abstraction of it.

TIME is VIKALPA,
it is an abstract, man-
made concept

DREAMS are VIKALPA
→ subconscious state
of mind

EVEN in
DEEP SLEEP brain activity DOES NOT
STOP (your breathing, digestion, etc...
is still operated)

the CONTENT of the mind
is absent.
the THOUGHTS still exist but
they are not present in
front of the MIND.

Yogis go to Samadhi,
normal people go to Sleep.
↳ SAMADHI & NIDRA are
similar as the both go to the
source, but in NIDRA, we are
not aware of it. In SAMADHI,
we are.

ASHTANGA YOGA → YOGA of EIGHT LIMBS

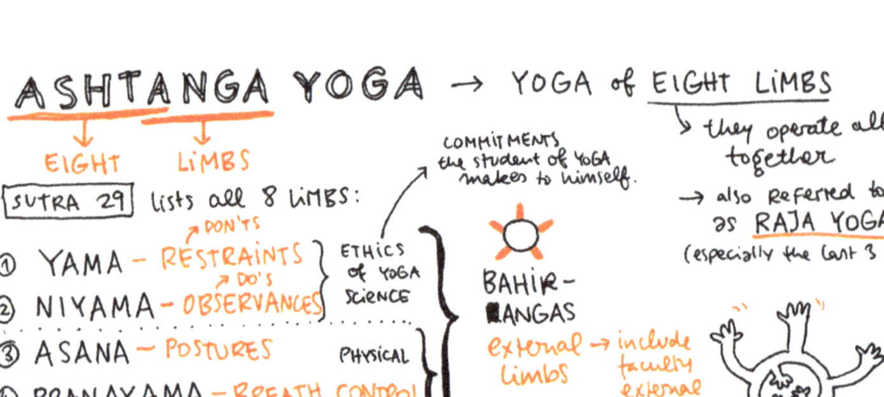

> they operate all together

→ also Referred to as **RAJA YOGA**
(especially the last 3 limbs)

EIGHT   LIMBS

SUTRA 29 | lists all 8 LIMBS:

COMMITMENTS the student of YOGA makes to himself.

① YAMA – RESTRAINTS → DON'TS
② NIYAMA – OBSERVANCES → DO'S } ETHICS OF YOGA SCIENCE

③ ASANA – POSTURES
④ PRANAYAMA – BREATH CONTROL
⑤ PRATYAHARA – WITHDRAWAL OF SENSES } PHYSICAL

⑥ DHARANA – CONCENTRATION
⑦ DHYANA – MEDITATION
⑧ SAMADHI – COGNITIVE SAMADHI
        – NON-COGNITIVE SAMADHI } SPIRITUAL

} MENTAL

BAHIR-RANGAS
external limbs → include faculty external to the mind

ANTAR-ANGAS
internal limbs → purely mental

YAMA

yama: to refrain / to regulate

→ YAMAS help to harmonize our relationship with the ONES AROUND US

– the VERY core of **YOGA**
↓
all other YAMAS & NIYAMAS are derived from & support

1. AHIMSA → NON-VIOLENCE
2. SATYA → TRUTHFULNESS
3. ASTEYA → NON-STEALING
4. BRAHMA-CHARYA → MODERATION
5. APARIGRAHA → NON-POSSESSING-NESS
= = =

AHIMSA
the ultimate truth.

AHIMSA is not only the ABSENCE of VIOLENCE but UNLIMITED, UN-CONDITIONAL LOVE

→ it's not the same as being COWARDLY!

The PURPOSE of all other YAMAS & NIYAMAS is to make your AHIMSA SPOTLESS.

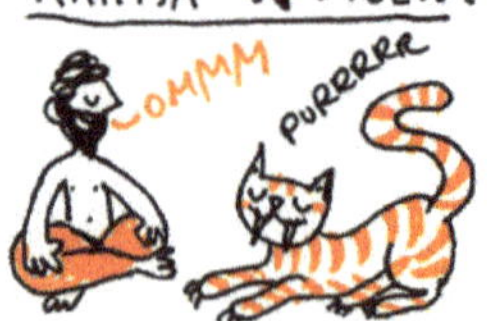

NIYAMA

the daily practices that we should do regularly

what can be observed when restrain is practiced

→ NIYAMAS help to harmonize with OURSELVES

1. SHAUCHA → CLEANLINESS
2. SANTOSHA → CONTENTMENT
3. TAPAH → AUSTERITY
4. SVADHYAYA → SELF-STUDY
5. ISVARAPRANI-DHANA → SURRENDE-RING to the SUPREME

Sarvatha – without limit of manner
Sarvada – without limit of time
Sarvabhutaram – not limited to any being
anabidroha – without the intention of inflicting any hurt or pain

AHIMSA is not inflicting pain in any way, at any time to any being

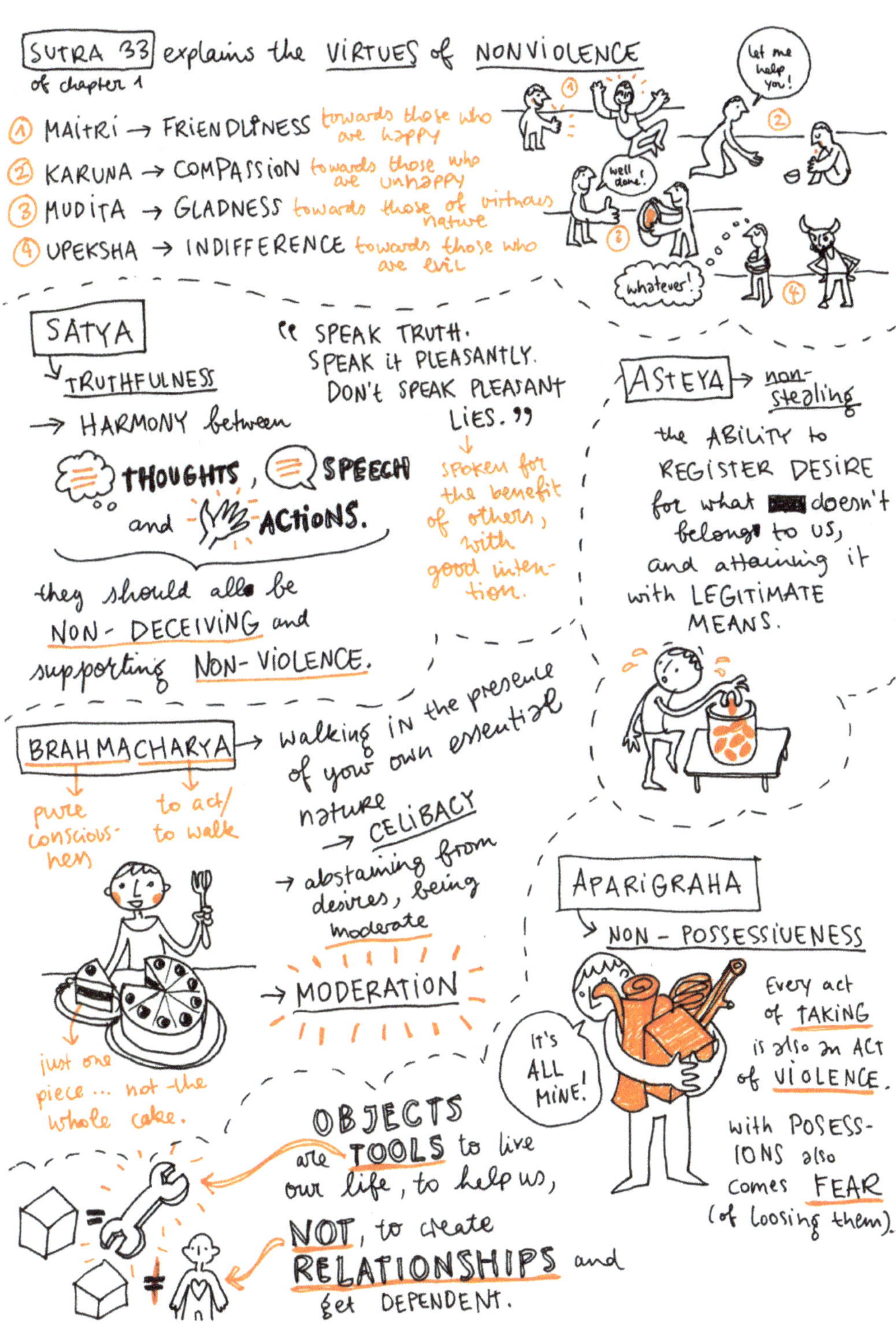

SUTRA 33 of chapter 1 explains the VIRTUES of NONVIOLENCE

1 MAITRI → FRIENDLINESS towards those who are happy
2 KARUNA → COMPASSION towards those who are unhappy
3 MUDITA → GLADNESS towards those of virtuous nature
4 UPEKSHA → INDIFFERENCE towards those who are evil

let me help you!
well done!
whatever!

SATYA
→ TRUTHFULNESS
→ HARMONY between
THOUGHTS, SPEECH and ACTIONS.
they should all be NON-DECEIVING and supporting NON-VIOLENCE.

"SPEAK TRUTH. SPEAK it PLEASANTLY. Don't SPEAK PLEASANT LIES."
spoken for the benefit of others, with good intention.

ASTEYA → non-stealing
the ABILITY to REGISTER DESIRE for what doesn't belong to us, and attaining it with LEGITIMATE MEANS.

BRAHMACHARYA
pure consciousness
to act/ to walk
walking in the presence of your own essential nature
→ CELIBACY
→ abstaining from desires, being moderate
→ MODERATION
just one piece ... not the whole cake.

APARIGRAHA
→ NON-POSSESSIVENESS
It's ALL MINE!
Every act of TAKING is also an ACT of VIOLENCE.
with POSESSIONS also comes FEAR (of loosing them).

OBJECTS are TOOLS to live our life, to help us, NOT, to create RELATIONSHIPS and get DEPENDENT.

NIYAMAS

SHAUCHA → CLEANLINESS

external
CLEANING our BODY, & CLEANING our EMOTIONS
internal
(by practising the virtues of NONVIOLENCE)

our BODY CONSTANTLY ACCUMULATES IMPURI-TIES & TOXINS
(& constantly oozes them)

→ These impurities distract us from deeper practice (e.g. a blocked nose makes it hard to MEDITATE)

OMMM → HMPF!

I will do it!

SANTOSHA
↳ CONTENTMENT
being happy with what we have and don't have.

but it's not indifference!

Everything is just fine as it is.

TAPAH
lit: generating the HEAT within
the heat of WILL.

WILLPOWER,
but without being violent towards yourself → be patient with yourself

INSPIRING yourself to CLIMB HIGHER, but also ACCEPTING the GROUNDS you are at.

SVADHYAYA
↳ SELF-STUDY
study be yourself
Realize yourself by applying what you learn.
WHATEVER we THINK, we BECOME.

ISHVARA PRANIDHANA
↳ SURRENDERING to the SUPREME

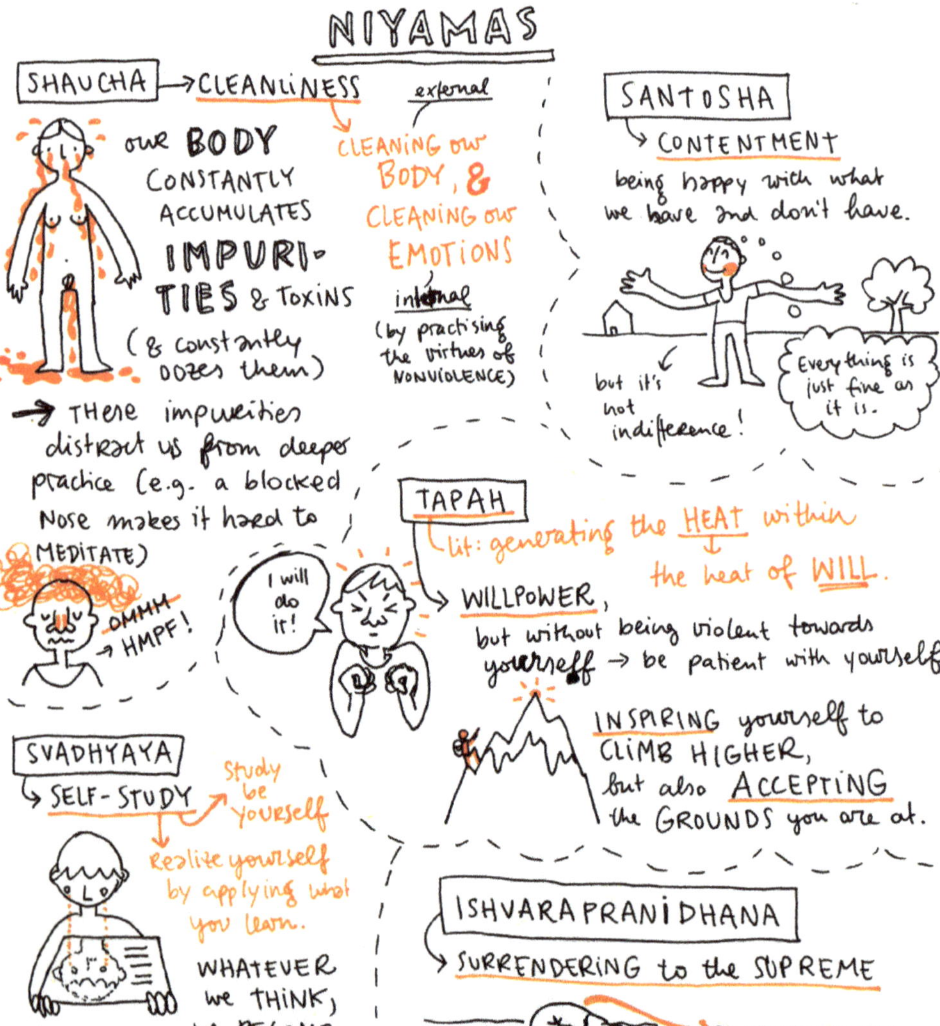

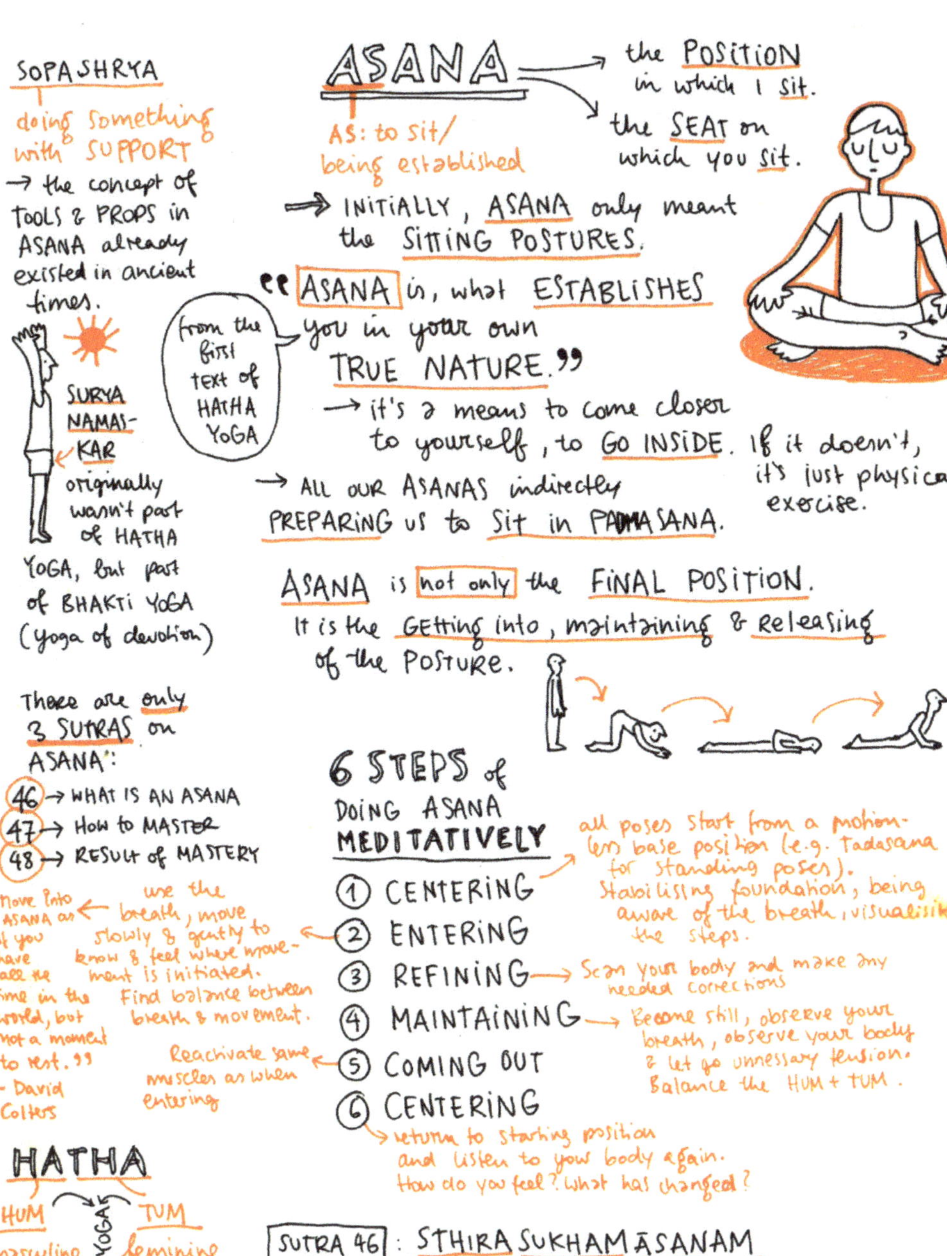

SOPASHRYA

doing something with **SUPPORT**
→ the concept of TOOLS & PROPS in ASANA already existed in ancient times.

SURYA NAMAS- KAR originally wasn't part of HATHA YOGA, but part of BHAKTI YOGA (yoga of devotion)

There are only **3 SUTRAS** on **ASANA:**
- (46) → WHAT IS AN ASANA
- (47) → HOW to MASTER
- (48) → RESULT of MASTERY

"Move into ASANA as if you have all the time in the world, but not a moment to rest." — David Colters

use the breath, move slowly & gently to know & feel where movement is initiated. Find balance between breath & movement.

Reactivate same muscles as when entering

ASANA → the POSITION in which I sit.
→ the SEAT on which you sit.

AS: to sit/ being established

→ INITIALLY, ASANA only meant the SITTING POSTURES.

" ASANA is, what ESTABLISHES you in your own TRUE NATURE. "

from the first text of HATHA YOGA

→ it's a means to come closer to yourself, to GO INSIDE. If it doesn't, it's just physical exercise.

→ ALL OUR ASANAS indirectly PREPARING us to sit in PADMASANA.

ASANA is not only the FINAL POSITION.
It is the GETTING into, maintaining & releasing of the POSTURE.

6 STEPS of DOING ASANA MEDITATIVELY

1. CENTERING
2. ENTERING
3. REFINING
4. MAINTAINING
5. COMING OUT
6. CENTERING

all poses start from a motion-less base position (e.g. Tadasana for standing poses). Stabilising foundation, being aware of the breath, visualising the steps.

→ Scan your body and make any needed corrections

→ Become still, observe your breath, observe your body & let go unnessary tension. Balance the HUM + TUM.

→ return to starting position and listen to your body again. How do you feel? What has changed?

HATHA

HUM masculine force, SUN, right side ↓ (Pingala) **ACTIVA-TION**

BALANCE these two = YOGA

TUM feminine force, MOON, left side ↓ (Ida) **RELAX-ATION**

SUTRA 46 : STHIRA SUKHAMĀSANAM

STEADY · COMFORTABLE/ EFFORT-LESS · BE ESTABLISHED

LEARNING and PRACTISING are TWO DIFFERENT THINGS.
→ the real learning comes from practise. Having learnt a posture is not the goal. Practising the ASANA is the goal.

experiencing!

THE POSTURE SHOULD BE STEADY & EFFORTLESS. (until it is that, you are still learning)

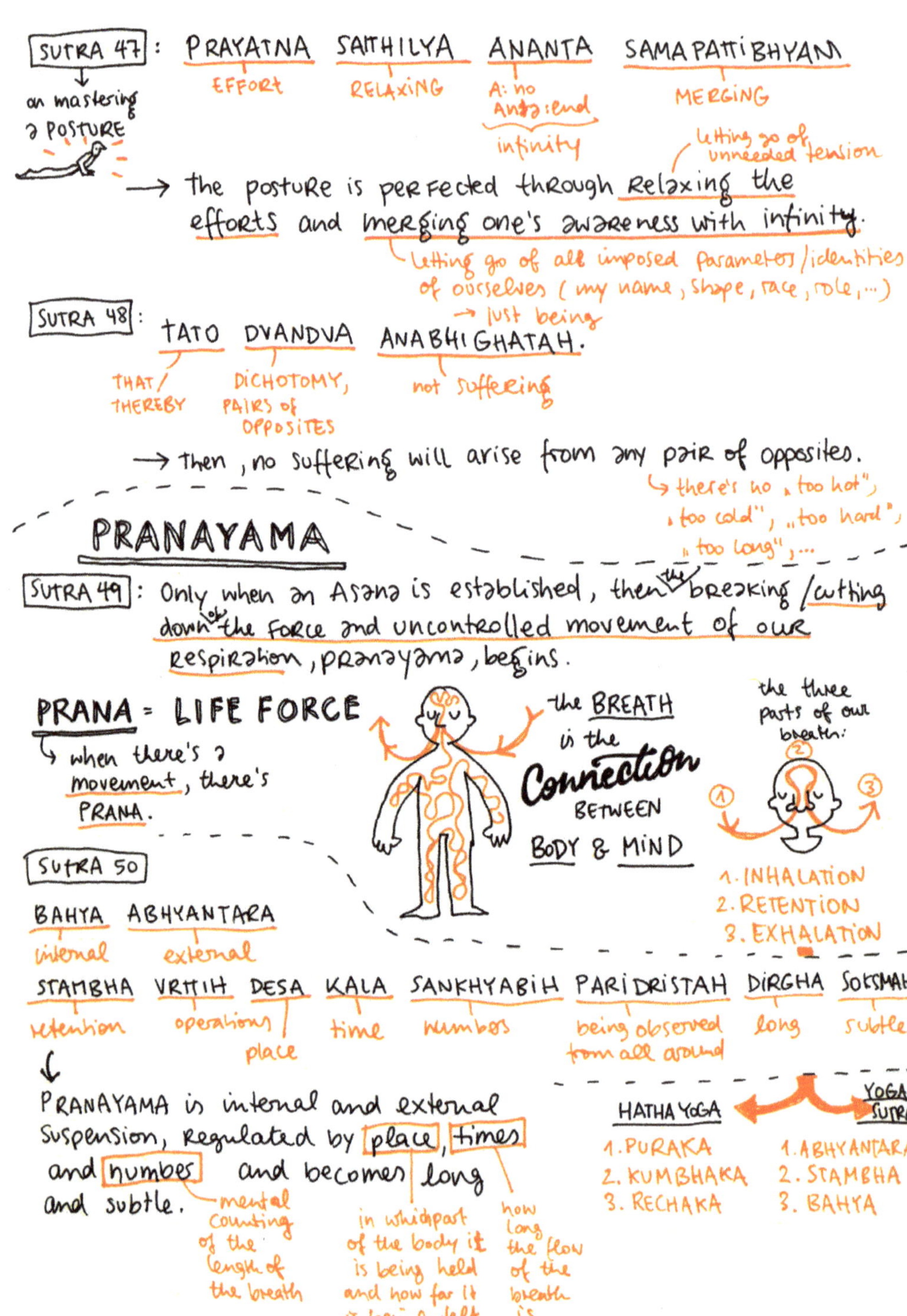

SUTRA 47: PRAYATNA SAITHILYA ANANTA SAMAPATTIBHYAM

- EFFORT
- RELAXING
- A: no / An(t)a:end / infinity
- MERGING — Letting go of unneeded tension

on mastering a POSTURE

→ the posture is perfected through Relaxing the efforts and merging one's awareness with infinity.

⌐ Letting go of all imposed parameters/identities of ourselves (my name, shape, race, role,...)
→ Just being

SUTRA 48: TATO DVANDVA ANABHIGHATAH.

- THAT / THEREBY
- DICHOTOMY, PAIRS OF OPPOSITES
- not suffering

→ Then, no suffering will arise from any pair of opposites.
⌐ there's no „too hot", „too cold", „too hard", „too long", ...

PRANAYAMA

SUTRA 49: Only when an Asana is established, then the breaking / cutting down the Force and uncontrolled movement of our respiration, pranayama, begins.

PRANA = LIFE FORCE
⌐ when there's a movement, there's PRANA.

the BREATH is the *Connection* BETWEEN BODY & MIND

the three parts of our breath:

1. INHALATION
2. RETENTION
3. EXHALATION

SUTRA 50

BAHYA ABHYANTARA
- internal
- external

STAMBHA VRTTIH DESA KALA SANKHYABIH PARIDRISTAH DIRGHA SUKSMAH
- retention
- operations / place
- time
- numbers
- being observed from all around
- long
- subtle

PRANAYAMA is internal and external Suspension, Regulated by [place], [times] and [numbers] and becomes [long] and subtle.

- mental counting of the length of the breath
- in which part of the body it is being held and how far it is being felt
- how long the flow of the breath is

HATHA YOGA	YOGA SUTRA
1. PURAKA	1. ABHYANTARA
2. KUMBHAKA	2. STAMBHA
3. RECHAKA	3. BAHYA

The CORRECT BREATHING is **DIAPHRAGMATIC** BREATHING
(≠ BELLY BREATHING)

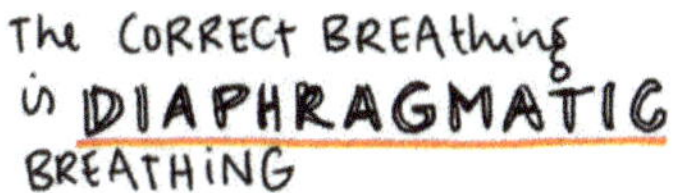

✔ "3-DIMENSIONAL"- BREATHING
→ you feel widening in the front, side & back.

→ only using the diaphragm,
✘ <u>NOT</u> the <u>INTERCOSTAL MUSCLES</u>

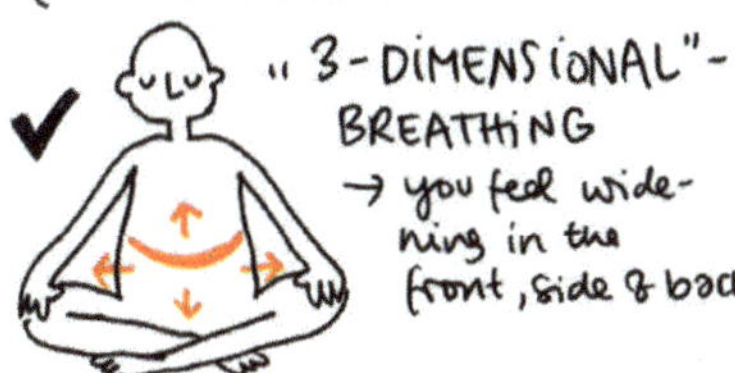

when inter-costal muscles are active, our nervous system activates fight-or-flight reaction.

the <u>PURPOSE</u> of PRANAYAMA is **KUMBHAKA** (Retention).

HATHA YOGA →

SAHITA KUMBHAKA
→ with FORCE
↓
holding the breath

→ SAHAJA KUMBHAKA
TRADITIONAL PRACTISES →
→ without FORCE / spontaneous
↓
"thinning" the breath by breathing slower & slower until breath ceases to be. (10, 5, 3, 2, 1 breaths per minute...)

NADI SHODANA is the "true" pranayama
→ work on this a lot.
→ make it long & subtle

<u>PRATYAHARA</u> → SENSE WITHDRAWAL

SUTRA 55: SVA VISHYA ASAMPRAYOGE CHITTA SVARUPA ANUKARA
own object disconnection mind-field own form/nature imitation

IVA INDRIYANAM PRATYAHARA.
as it were of senses sense withdrawal

when the senses are disconnected from the object, thereby the mind has become stabilised & the <u>senses</u> imitate the steadiness, stability and calmness of mind, that is PRATYAHARA.

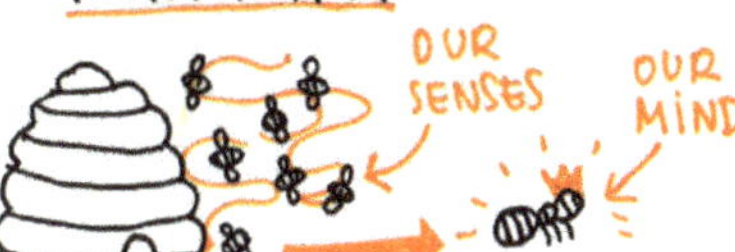

when you want to MOVE a BEEHIVE, Don't try to move a single bee at a time. You try to <u>MOVE</u> the <u>QUEEN BEE</u> and ALL the BEES will <u>follow</u>!

→ when the MIND becomes STILL, the SENSES will <u>follow</u>.

DHARANA → CONCENTRATION

DESHA BANDHAH CHITTASYA DHARANA
place to tie up/ bind of mind concentration

To tie up the mind in one particular <u>place</u> is called concentration.

external: e.g. a candle ← sound or images (mantra)
internal: e.g. a chakra

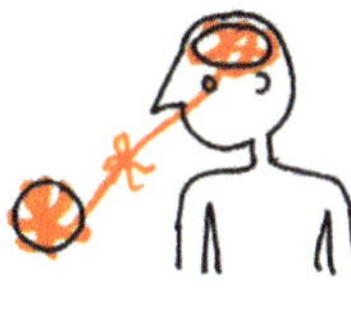

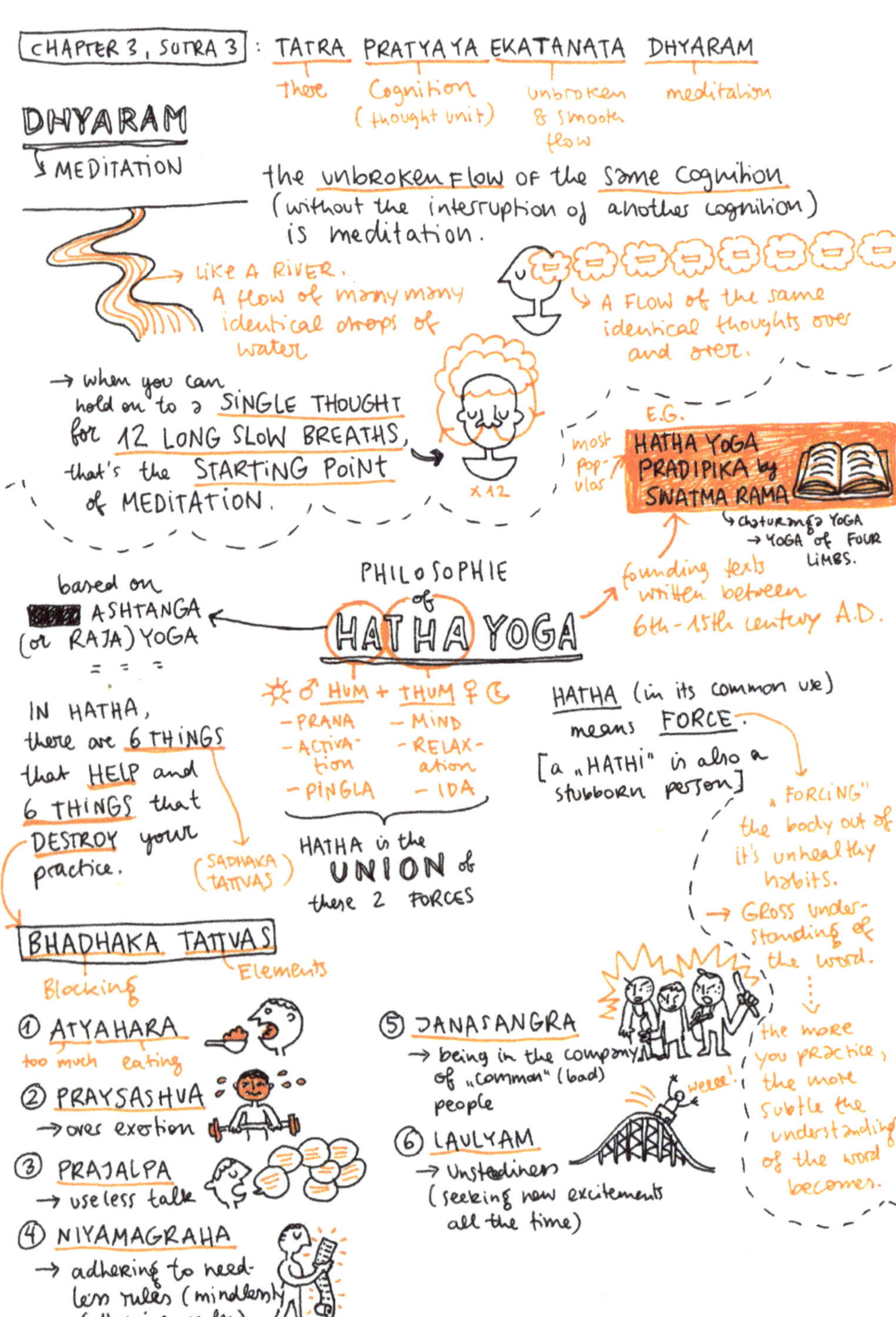

CHAPTER 3, SUTRA 3 : TATRA PRATYAYA EKATANATA DHYARAM
there   Cognition   unbroken   meditation
(thought unit)   & smooth
flow

DHYARAM
↳ MEDITATION

the unbroken FLOW of the same Cognition
(without the interruption of another cognition)
is meditation.

→ LIKE A RIVER.
A flow of many many
identical drops of
water

↳ A FLOW of the same
identical thoughts over
and over.

→ when you can
hold on to a SINGLE THOUGHT
for 12 LONG SLOW BREATHS,
that's the STARTING POINT
of MEDITATION.

× 12

E.G.
most
pop-
ular
HATHA YOGA
PRADIPIKA by
SWATMA RAMA
↳ chaturanga Yoga
→ YOGA of FOUR
LIMBS.

founding texts
written between
6th - 15th century A.D.

PHILOSOPHIE
of
HATHA YOGA

based on
ASHTANGA
(or RAJA) YOGA
= = =

☼ ♂ HUM + THUM ♀ ☾
- PRANA   - MIND
- ACTIVA-   - RELAX-
tion   ation
- PINGLA   - IDA

HATHA (in its common use)
means FORCE.
[a "HATHI" is also a
stubborn person]

"FORCING"
the body out of
it's unhealthy
habits.
→ GROSS under-
standing of
the word.

IN HATHA,
there are 6 THINGS
that HELP and
6 THINGS that
DESTROY your
practice.

SADHAKA
TATTVAS

HATHA is the
UNION of
these 2 FORCES

the more
you practice,
the more
subtle the
understanding
of the word
becomes.

BHADHAKA TATTVAS
Blocking   Elements

① ATYAHARA
too much eating

② PRAYSASHVA
→ over exertion

③ PRAJALPA
→ useless talk

④ NIYAMAGRAHA
→ adhering to need-
less rules (mindlessly
following rules)

⑤ JANASANGRA
→ being in the company
of "common" (bad)
people

⑥ LAULYAM
→ Unsteadiness
(seeking new excitements
all the time)

weee!

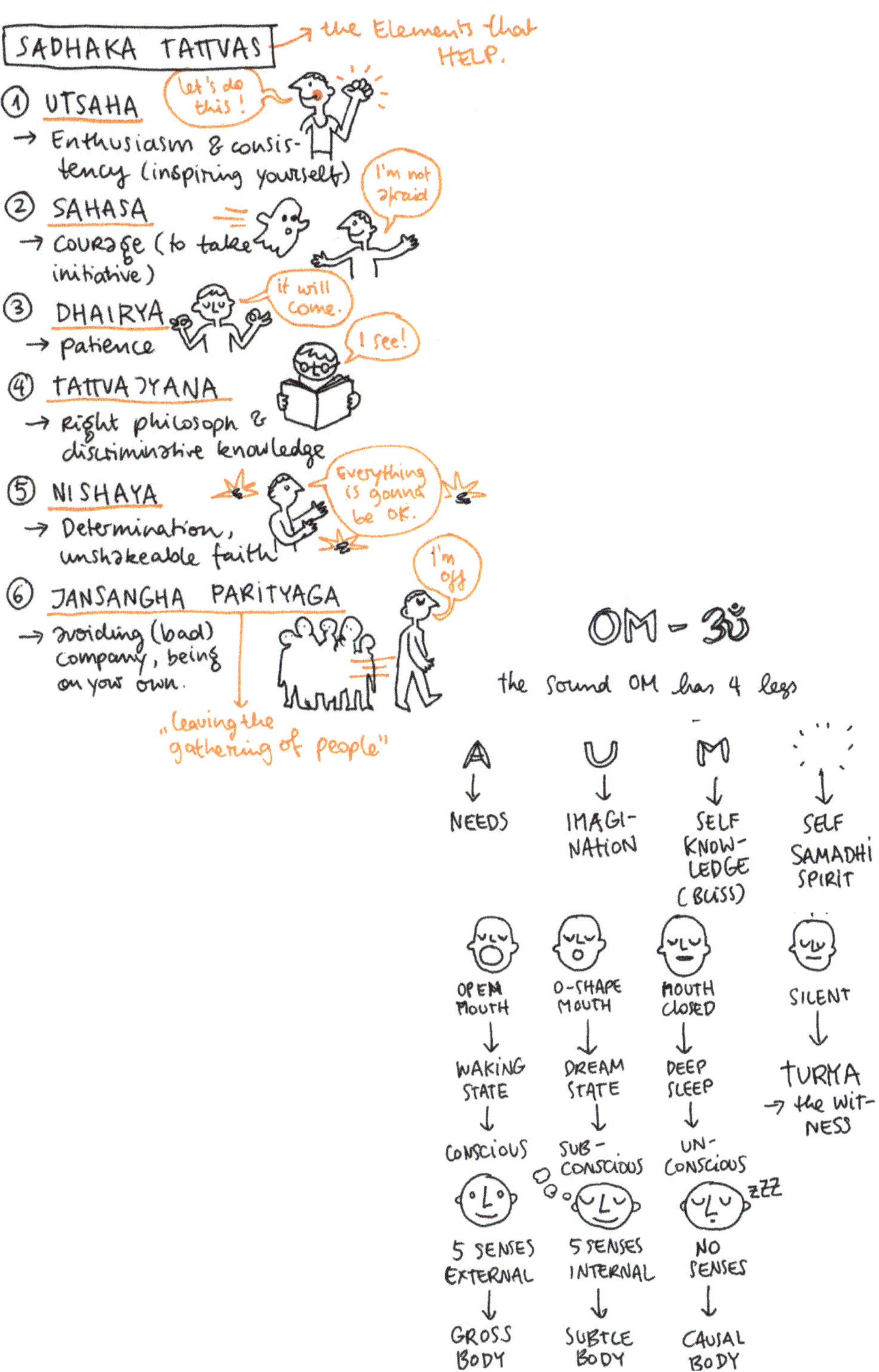

SADHAKA TATTVAS → the Elements that HELP.

① UTSAHA
→ Enthusiasm & consistency (inspiring yourself)
let's do this!

② SAHASA
→ courage (to take initiative)
I'm not afraid

③ DHAIRYA
→ patience
it will come.

④ TATTVA JYANA
→ right philosoph & discriminative knowledge
I see!

⑤ NISHAYA
→ Determination, unshakeable faith
Everything is gonna be OK.

⑥ JANSANGHA PARITYAGA
→ avoiding (bad) company, being on your own.
I'm off
"leaving the gathering of people"

OM - ॐ
the sound OM has 4 legs

A → NEEDS
U → IMAGINATION
M → SELF KNOWLEDGE (BLISS)
→ SELF SAMADHI SPIRIT

OPEN MOUTH
O-SHAPE MOUTH
MOUTH CLOSED
SILENT

WAKING STATE
DREAM STATE
DEEP SLEEP
TURYA → the witness

CONSCIOUS
SUB-CONSCIOUS
UN-CONSCIOUS

5 SENSES EXTERNAL
5 SENSES INTERNAL
NO SENSES

GROSS BODY
SUBTLE BODY
CAUSAL BODY

ABOUT THE AUTHOR

EVA-LOTTA LAMM IS A UX DESIGNER, ILLUSTRATOR AND
VISUAL THINKER. SHE GREW UP IN GERMANY, WORKED IN
PARIS AND LONDON FOR A FEW YEARS BEFORE PACKING
UP HER BACKPACK AND TRAVELLING THE WORLD FOR 14
MONTHS. AFTER BEING A (SEMI-)NOMAD FOR OVER TWO
YEARS, SHE IS NOW BASED AS AN INDEPENDENT DESIGNER
IN BERLIN.

BESIDES HER DESIGN WORK, SHE HAS BEEN TAKING
SKETCHNOTES AT HUNDREDS OF TALKS AND CONFERENCES.
DURING HER WORLD TRIP, SHE DOCUMENTED HER
EXPERIENCE AS DAILY SKETCHNOTES IN HER TRAVEL DIARY.

IN HER PERSONAL SKETCHING PRACTICE, SHE IS EXPLORING
THE AREA OF VISUAL IMPROVISATION, WHERE SHE IS
LOOKING AT THE PARALLELS BETWEEN SKETCHING AND
IMPROVISATION AND EXPERIMENTS WITH HOW THE
PRINCIPLES FROM HER REGULAR THEATER IMPROVISATION
PRACTICE CAN BE USED TO INSPIRE VISUAL WORK.

FIND OUT MORE ABOUT EVA-LOTTA's WORK:
WWW.EVALOTTA.NET
WWW.EVALOTTA.SHOP

TWITTER / INSTAGRAM / FLICKR:
@EVALOTTCHEN

SURYA NAMASKAR A

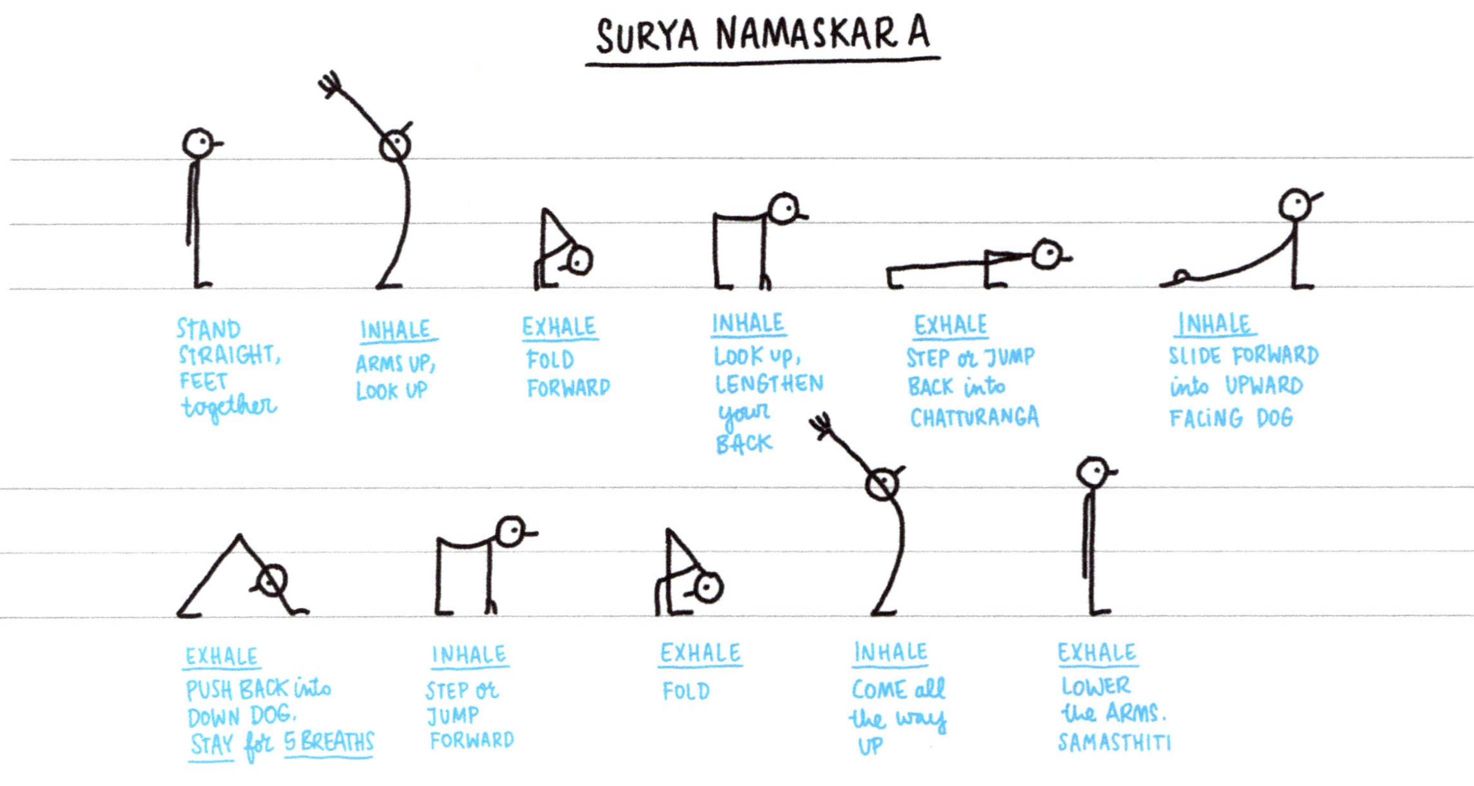

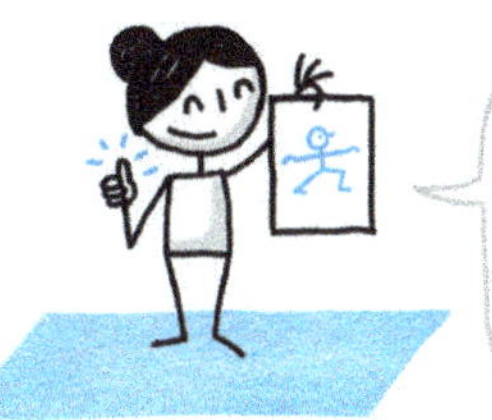

THE

YOGANOTES BOOK

CAN SHOW you HOW!

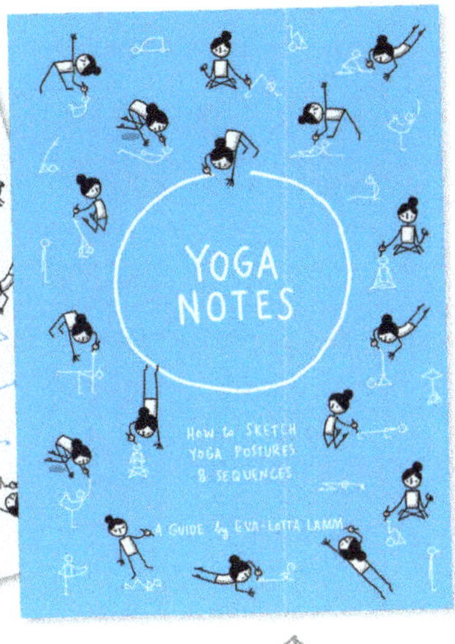

AVAILABLE as E-BOOK or PRINTED BOOK

BASIC PRINCIPLES of SKETCHING YOGA Stick FIGURES

&

STEP-BY-STEP INSTRUCTIONS for over 80 ASANAS & their VARIATIONS

for PRACTITIONERS

CAPTURE your FAVOURITE CLASSES

CREATE a personalized HOME PRACTICE PLAN

for TEACHERS

PLAN your own CLASSES

for TEACHER TRAINEES

TAKE NOTES during your TEACHER TRAINING COURSE

WWW.YOGANOTES.NET

WWW.YOGANOTES.DE

DEUTSCHE VERSION

WWW.EVALOTTA.SHOP/YOGA

@EVALOTTCHEN

BERLIN · 2017